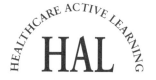

HEALTHCARE ACTIVE LEARNING

HAL

PHYSIOLOGY

Start date

Target completion date

Tutor for this topic

Contact number

USING THIS WORKBOOK

The workbook is divided into 'Sessions', covering specific subjects.

In the introduction to each learning pack there is a learner profile to help you assess your current knowledge of the subjects covered in each session.

Each session has clear learning objectives. They indicate what you will be able to achieve or learn by completing that session.

Each session has a summary to remind you of the key points of the subjects covered.

Each session contains text, diagrams and learning activities that relate to the stated objectives.

It is important to complete each activity, making your own notes and writing in answers in the space provided. **Remember this is your own workbook—you are allowed to write on it**.

Now try an example activity.

ACTIVITY

This activity shows you what happens when cells work without oxygen. This really is a physical activity, so please only try it if you are fully fit.

First, raise one arm straight up in the air above your head, and let the other hand rest by your side. Clench both fists tightly, and then open out your fingers wide. Repeat this at the rate of once or twice a second. Try to keep clenching both fists at the same rate. Keep going for about five minutes, and record what you observe.

Stop and rest for a minute. Then try again, with the opposite arm raised this time. Again, record your observations.

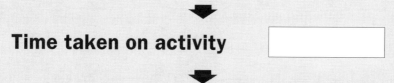

Suggested timings are given for each activity. These are only a guide. You may like to note how long it took you to complete this activity, as it may help in planning the time needed for working through the sessions.

Time taken on activity

Time management is important. While we recognise that people learn at different speeds, this pack is designed to take 20 study hours (your tutor will also advise you). You should allocate time during each week for study.

Take some time now to identify likely periods that you can set aside for study during the week.

	Mon	Tues	Wed	Thurs	Fri	Sat	Sun
am							
pm							
eve							

At the end of the learning pack, there is a learning review to help you assess whether you have achieved the learning objectives.

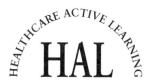

PHYSIOLOGY

Stephen W. Ashurst BSc PhD RGN

Staff Nurse (Intensive Care) and Part-time Lecturer,
Department of Advanced Nursing Studies, North East Wales Institute

Jenny Coe BA MA Cert Ed SRN DipNurse (Lond) RNT

Senior Lecturer, Department of Advanced Nursing Studies,
North East Wales Institute

Patricia A. Lyne BSc PhD RGN

Reader in Nursing Research, Department of Advanced Nursing,
The North East Wales Institute

THE OPEN LEARNING FOUNDATION

CHURCHILL LIVINGSTONE

EDINBURGH LONDON MADRID MELBOURNE NEW YORK AND TOKYO 1995

CHURCHILL LIVINGSTONE
Medical Division of Longman Group UK Limited

Distributed in the United States of America by Churchill
Livingstone Inc., 650 Avenue of the Americas, New York,
N.Y. 10011, and by associated companies, branches and
representatives throughout the world.

First published 1995

ISBN 0 443 05274 3

British Library of Cataloguing in Publication Data
A catalogue record for this book is available from the
British Library.

Library of Congress Cataloging in Publication Data
A catalogue record for this book is available from the
Library of Congress

Printed and bound by Bell and Bain Ltd., Glasgow

For The Open Learning Foundation

Director of Programmes: Leslie Mapp
Series Editor: Robert Adams
Programmes Manager: Kathleen Farren
Production Manager: Steve Moulds

For Churchill Livingstone

Director (NAH): Peter Shepherd
Project Development Editor: Mairi McCubbin
Project Manager: Valerie Burgess
Design Direction: Judith Wright
Pre-press Project Manager: Neil Dickson
Pre-press Desktop Operator: Kate Walshaw
Sales Promotion Executive: Hilary Brown

Contents

OPEN LEARNING
FOUNDATION
TEAM MEMBERS

Writers: Dr Stephen W. Ashurst
Staff Nurse (Intensive Care) and Part-time Lecturer,
Department of Advanced Nursing Studies, North East Wales Institute

Jenny Coe
Senior Lecturer, Department of Advanced Nursing Studies,
North East Wales Institute

Dr Patricia A. Lyne
Reader in Nursing Research, Department of Advanced Nursing,
The North East Wales Institute

Editors: Bruce Gilham
Managing Director, Form Word Ltd

Dr Elisabeth Clarke
Distance Learning Programme Coordinator,
Royal College of Nursing

Reviewers: Professor Justus Akinsaya
Pro Vice Chancellor, International Development,
Anglia Polytechnic University

John Mears
Queen Charlotte's College of Health and Science

Series Editor: Robert Adams
OLF Programme Head,
Social Work and Health and Nursing,
University of Humberside

THE OPEN LEARNING FOUNDATION

Higher education has grown considerably in recent years. As well as catering for more students, universities are facing the challenge of providing for an increasingly diverse student population. Students have a wider range of backgrounds and previous educational qualifications. There are greater numbers of mature students. There is a greater need for part-time courses and continuing education and professional development programmes.

The Open Learning Foundation helps over 20 member institutions meet this growing and diverse demand – through the production of high-quality teaching and learning materials, within a strategy of creating a framework for more flexible learning. It offers member institutions the capability to increase their range of teaching options and to cover subjects in greater breadth and depth.

It does not enrol its own students. Rather, The Open Learning Foundation, by developing and promoting the greater use of open and distance learning, enables universities and others in higher education to make study more accessible and cost-effective for individual students and for business through offering more choice and more flexible courses.

Formed in 1990, the Foundation's policy objectives are to:

- improve the quality of higher education and training

- increase the quantity of higher education and training

- raise the efficiency of higher education and training delivery.

In working to meet these objectives, The Open Learning Foundation develops new teaching and learning materials, encourages and facilitates more and better staff development, and promotes greater responsiveness to change within higher education institutions. The Foundation works in partnership with its members and other higher education bodies to develop new approaches to teaching and learning.

In developing new teaching and learning materials, the Foundation has:

- a track record of offering customers a swift and flexible response

- a national network of members able to provide local support and guidance

- the ability to draw on significant national expertise in producing and delivering open learning

- complete freedom to seek out the best writers, materials and resources to secure development.

INTRODUCTION

Where this unit fits in

This unit is part of a series which deals with the biological sciences from the point of view of health care professionals. The others are Genetics and Biochemistry.

Genetics concerns the way in which characteristics are passed on from parents to children. These characteristics are controlled through the genetic material which each living cell contains.

Biochemistry deals with the immediate effects of the genetic composition of the cells – the way that chemicals are organised and used by the cells to carry out the processes which constitute 'life'.

Physiology takes a wider view of the body. This science deals with the way in which collections of cells are organised to form organs such as the heart and liver, and the way in which these organs work together in the body. Many physiological processes are readily observable, but it is important to remember that they depend upon underlying biochemical and genetic activities which can only be identified in the laboratory.

The unit is written so that it can be studied independently. We do not assume that you have studied the other units. Where material from these units is helpful, extracts are provided in the Resource section. However, if you intend to study all three units it is best to work through them in the order indicated above – i.e. Genetics, then Biochemistry, then Physiology.

The relevance of physiology to nursing practice

Physiology deals with the way that the various systems of the body work to produce the activities which we recognise as living; for example, the way that the digestive system operates so that we can eat and obtain nutrition. Understanding the way that the systems work in health and illness is very important for the delivery of nursing care.

Even more importantly, physiology emphasises the interaction between these systems, and the way that their activities are adjusted to keep the body functioning as well as possible. Nurses work with people to help them make the most of their bodies' natural physiological capacity to cope with change and to recover from illness. So physiology has a very close and direct link with nursing.

Finally, physiology is concerned with the way that the body achieves a state of balance, despite all the changes that happen daily. It enables us to understand what happens when imbalance occurs and how health care aims to restore balance. In fact, the basic principles of physiology are very similar to those nursing models which emphasise the nurse's role in assisting people to regain wellbeing.

The scope of this unit

This is an open learning unit. Open learning (OL) is essentially an active process.

It requires you to be actively engaged with the OL materials, thinking about questions and exploring topics for yourself. You should allow about 20 hours for your study of this material, including the time that you spend on the activities.

So this is not a textbook to be read from cover to cover. There are excellent, comprehensive textbooks on physiology that you may go on to read. These are usually structured around the twelve major systems of the body. This unit is rather different in that it does not try to cover all the systems or to deal with the whole of physiology. Instead, it takes a major theme of importance to nurses and follows it through to illustrate some of the most important principles of the subject that nurses need to understand in order to inform their practice.

We make no assumptions about your previous knowledge of the subject, so you can study the unit even if you have not done any biology at all.

How to use this unit

As you read the text you will find suggestions about various kinds of things to do. These activities are an important part of the learning process, so please don't be tempted to skip over them.

LEARNING PROFILE

Below is a list of learning outcomes for each session in this unit. You can use it to identify your current familiarity with the subject, and so to consider how the unit can help you to develop your knowledge and understanding. The list is not intended to cover all the details discussed in every session, and so the learning profile should only be used for general guidance.

For each of the learning outcomes listed below, tick the box that corresponds most closely to your own abilities. This will provide you with an assessment of your current understanding and confidence in the areas that you will study in this unit.

	Not at all	Partly	Quite well	Very well
Session One				
I can:				
• explain, in general terms, the relevance of physiological principles to the delivery of nursing care	☐	☐	☐	☐
• describe the volume and distribution of fluid in the human body	☐	☐	☐	☐
• explain the idea of water balance	☐	☐	☐	☐
• outline the function of intercellular fluid in providing a stable internal environment	☐	☐	☐	☐
• describe the effects of fluid deprivation on the human body	☐	☐	☐	☐
• define the term 'oedema'	☐	☐	☐	☐
• describe the forces which result in the formation of intercellular fluid	☐	☐	☐	☐

	Not at all	Partly	Quite well	Very well

- explain the consequences of an imbalance in these forces ☐ ☐ ☐ ☐
- predict what will happen if any one of these forces, for example, the osmotic pressure of the plasma, changes drastically ☐ ☐ ☐ ☐
- define the term homeostasis and understand what it means in relation to the body's fluid balance ☐ ☐ ☐ ☐
- outline the principles underlying the nursing care of a person with peripheral oedema. ☐ ☐ ☐ ☐

Session Two

I can:

- outline the structure of the normal kidney and the way in which urine is produced ☐ ☐ ☐ ☐
- explain the effects of reduced fluid intake ☐ ☐ ☐ ☐
- explain why fluids are given, as a matter of urgency, to casualties who have suffered blood loss ☐ ☐ ☐ ☐
- describe the role of the kidney in the homeostatic processes which regulate BP ☐ ☐ ☐ ☐
- explain the principle of feedback control as it applies to the renin/angiotensin system ☐ ☐ ☐ ☐
- describe and explain the symptoms of chronic and acute renal failure ☐ ☐ ☐ ☐
- discuss the role of the clinical nurse specialist working in a renal unit ☐ ☐ ☐ ☐
- outline the relationship between renal and cardiac function. ☐ ☐ ☐ ☐

Session Three

I can:

- describe, in outline, the structure and function of the heart ☐ ☐ ☐ ☐
- identify the way in which blood flows through the heart to the lungs and the rest of the body ☐ ☐ ☐ ☐
- explain the way that the heart beat is initiated and apply this understanding to supporting patients undergoing electrocardiogram investigations ☐ ☐ ☐ ☐
- describe how the heart rate is varied to meet the changing needs of the body ☐ ☐ ☐ ☐
- explain how variations in the heart beat contribute to the maintenance of homeostasis ☐ ☐ ☐ ☐
- explain the relationship between the activity of the heart and the blood pressure ☐ ☐ ☐ ☐
- identify the effects of right- and left-sided heart failure ☐ ☐ ☐ ☐

	Not at all	Partly	Quite well	Very well
• explain how oedema may be caused by heart failure	☐	☐	☐	☐
• outline the relationship between the cardiovascular and respiratory systems.	☐	☐	☐	☐

Session Four

I can:

	Not at all	Partly	Quite well	Very well
• describe what happens during normal breathing, including the respiratory movements and the exchange of gases at the lung surface	☐	☐	☐	☐
• explain the effects of breathing difficulty, in general terms	☐	☐	☐	☐
• outline the structure and characteristics of the lungs	☐	☐	☐	☐
• describe how the rate of breathing is controlled	☐	☐	☐	☐
• understand the effects of lung damage on the pulmonary and systemic circulation	☐	☐	☐	☐
• give an account, in outline only, of the role of histamine in the normal response to damage and in anaphylaxis	☐	☐	☐	☐
• discuss the nature of asthma and its effects on people	☐	☐	☐	☐
• use my understanding of physiology to suggest how nurses can best support people with asthma and other breathing problems.	☐	☐	☐	☐

Session Five

I can:

	Not at all	Partly	Quite well	Very well
• describe the role of the thyroid hormones in the control of temperature	☐	☐	☐	☐
• discuss the contribution of the nervous and hormonal systems to the maintenance of temperature homeostasis	☐	☐	☐	☐
• explain how heatstroke, pyrexia and hypothermia are brought about	☐	☐	☐	☐
• outline the regular manner in which body temperature varies during the day	☐	☐	☐	☐
• apply my knowledge of variations in body temperature to the provision of care.	☐	☐	☐	☐

Session Six

I can:

	Not at all	Partly	Quite well	Very well
• describe how adrenaline is produced and affects several body systems	☐	☐	☐	☐
• outline the relationship between adrenaline and the sympathetic nervous system	☐	☐	☐	☐

	Not at all	Partly	Quite well	Very well
• explain how a nerve impulse travels along a nerve fibre	☐	☐	☐	☐
• outline how neurotransmitters work	☐	☐	☐	☐
• draw a simple diagram of a neuron				
• recognise the signs which show that a person is afraid				
• identify the causes of 'everyday' pain	☐	☐	☐	☐
• describe how referred pain is caused	☐	☐	☐	☐
• explain how painful stimuli can be modified in the nervous system	☐	☐	☐	☐
• outline the role of the nurse in caring for people suffering from acute and chronic pain	☐	☐	☐	☐
• relate the possible consequences of prolonged stress to patient care.	☐	☐	☐	☐

Session One

Water everywhere

Session objectives

When you have completed this introductory session you should be able to:

- explain, in general terms, the relevance of physiological principles to the delivery of nursing care

- describe the volume and distribution of fluid in the human body

- explain the idea of water balance

- outline the function of intercellular fluid in providing a stable internal environment

- describe the effects of fluid deprivation on the human body

- define the term 'oedema'

- describe the forces which result in the formation of intercellular fluid

- explain the consequences of an imbalance in these forces

- predict what will happen if any one of these forces, for example, the osmotic pressure of the plasma, changes drastically

- define the term homeostasis and understand what it means in relation to the body's fluid balance

- outline the principles underlying the nursing care of a person with peripheral oedema.

1: Fluids in the right places

Water: a very special liquid

We begin this unit by considering the fluid component of the human body. A great deal of nursing activity is concerned with ensuring that people in their care are well **hydrated** – in other words that, whatever their circumstances, they have the right amount of fluid in their bodies. This is one of the most valuable ways in which nurses can assist people who are not able to care for themselves. Another major concern of nurses and other health carers relates to the problems people experience when fluid accumulates in the wrong place. Displaced fluid results in some very troublesome symptoms – a condition known as **oedema**. This unit therefore begins by considering how fluid is usually distributed, and then explores what happens when fluids accumulate in the wrong places.

All the fluid in the body is based on water. This liquid is so familiar that we tend to take it very much for granted (at least as long as it is plentiful) and think of it as nothing special. However, this is far from the case, because water is like no other liquid. It has unique properties which make life as we know it possible.

How much water?

Many people who have not studied the biological sciences have no idea how much water their body contains. We asked a number of non-medical friends and relatives and got answers ranging from 5% to 95%. The first activity in this unit is designed to refresh your own memory of the actual volume of water in the body. We would like you to do this in order to form a mental picture of this volume, as an aid to understanding the importance of water.

ACTIVITY 1   ALLOW **3** MINUTES

Please read the following paragraph and carry out the calculation at the end.

The amount of fluid in the body makes a significant contribution to its weight. Approximately 60% of the body is water under normal conditions. This percentage goes up and down according to external conditions and one of the ways that crash diets work is by temporarily removing some of this water – producing an apparent weight loss. Using the approximate figure of 60%, see if you can calculate the amount of water in your own body, in litres. One litre of water weighs one kilogram. Record your answer in the space below.

Commentary

If your weight is about 70 kg (10 stones) the amount of water in your body is 42 litres. If you weigh more or less than this, you can easily find the amount of water by using the equation:

Vol. of body water (litres) = $\dfrac{\text{Body weight (kg)} \times 60}{100}$

In order to form a mental picture of this volume of water it may help to note that an ordinary household bucket holds approximately 8 litres.

Inputs and outputs

The water content of the body is in a dynamic state – in other words it is constantly changing and being renewed, even though the total amount remains roughly the same. A simple analogy for this is a pond with a stream flowing through it. The level in the pond remains constant, but the water it contains is constantly changing. This pond is in a dynamic equilibrium.

This concept applies to most of the constituents of the body. Even seemingly permanent structures like bones are in a constant state of change. The materials in them are constantly being renewed. However, it is much easier to observe the dynamic state of water in the body because we can actually observe many of the inputs and outputs; whereas we are not aware that, for example, minerals are constantly being replaced in our bones.

ACTIVITY 2 ALLOW 5 MINUTES

- Think about the ways in which you take water into your body. Make a list of these in column 1 of *Table 1* below.
- Next, consider the ways in which you lose water from the body. List these in column 2 of the same table.
- Finally, thinking about your own way of life, can you estimate how much you gain and lose in these ways over an average 24 hour period? If so, make a note of your estimates in columns 1a and 2a.

Column 1	1a	2	2a

Table 1 Water inputs and outputs

Commentary

Here is the table filled in. I wonder how close your estimates came to the figures here?

Inputs	Volume	Outputs	Volume
Drinking	1.2 litres	Urine	1.5 litres
Food	1.0 litres	Faeces	0.1 litres
The body's own activity (metabolism)	0.35 litres	Evaporation from skin and lungs	0.9 litres
		Sweat	0.05 litres
Total	2.55 litres		2.55 litres

Table 2 Activity 1 completed

The important things to notice about this table are:

- the total inputs and outputs are the same
- the amount of water that is changed during 24 hours is 2.55 litres, that is, approximately $\frac{1}{20}$ of the total water in the body.

This information shows that, under normal circumstances, the body is in **water balance** – the inputs and outputs are the same. This is a dynamic state, because the water is continually being renewed.

Body fluids

The water in the body is not simply spread around evenly, as it would be if absorbed into a very large sponge. Some is inside the cells (forming the basis of **intracellular fluids**), and some outside (forming the basis of the **extracellular fluids**). The fluid outside the cells is composed mainly of blood plasma and the fluid between and around the cells (**intercellular** or **interstitial** fluid). *Figures 1a* and *1b* show this in a diagrammatic form. In *Figure 1a* the location of these three different types of fluid is illustrated. *Figure 1b* shows their different relative volumes.

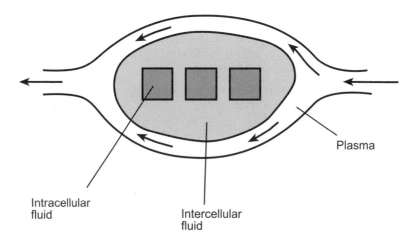

Figure 1a The relationship between body fluids

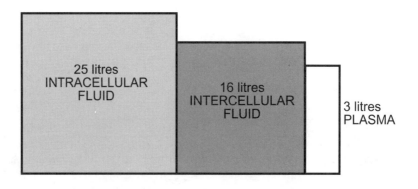

Figure 1b Relative volumes of body fluid

Figure 1b shows the approximate volumes of the three body fluids in a person with a lean body. The amount of body fluid is related to the lean mass of the body – that is, the total weight less the weight of stored fat.

In a healthy person, body fluids are distributed as shown here. They are 'in the right places'. When people are unwell, their problems often arise from changes in fluid volume and from fluid being wrongly distributed around the body. We will be looking at this closely later. First we need to look at the various kinds of body fluid in more detail in order to understand the relationship between them, and the way this contributes to the body's normal function.

Keeping the environment constant

Figure 1a was deliberately drawn as a set of interlocking compartments to emphasise that the intercellular fluid surrounds the fluid in the cells. This fluid acts as a **buffer** between the vulnerable living cells and the external environment, which is continually changing.

The term 'buffer' has a technical meaning in physiology which can be partly understood if we consider the use of the term on the railways. Here the buffers are designed to *absorb the impact* if the train rams into the end of the line. In the same sense, the intercellular fluid absorbs the impact of the changes outside the body and prevents them from having drastic effects on the cells inside. This protective action is possible because the body contains mechanisms for adjusting the composition of the fluid surrounding the cells in response to any changes that occur. So while the composition of the plasma may change considerably from time to time, the composition of the intercellular fluid is kept constant, thus acting as a buffer zone between the plasma and the living cells.

The buffering action is made possible because the different fluids have different substances dissolved in them. The differences are shown in *Table 3*.

DISSOLVED SUBSTANCES	INTRACELLULAR FLUID	EXTRACELLULAR FLUIDS	
		INTERCELLULAR	PLASMA
Potassium	+ + + +	+	+
Sodium	+	+ + + +	+ + + +
Protein	+ +	+	+ + +
Magnesium	+ +	trace	+
Phosphate	+ + + +	trace	+ +
Chlorine	+	+ +	+ +
Bicarbonate		+	+

Table 3 Composition of body fluids

One of the main differences between the various body fluids is that plasma and the intracellular fluid contain more protein than the intercellular fluid. Later you will see why this is important. The intercellular fluid represents the environment of the cells and, just as our environment determines our wellbeing, the intercellular fluid influences the wellbeing of the living cells. By its buffering action, this fluid creates a constant environment for the cells. So it is important that it provides the right environment as far as possible. In particular, its chemical composition needs to remain constant, even though the inputs of water and other substances to the body as a whole vary greatly throughout the day.

ACTIVITY 3

To illustrate how this environment is kept constant, imagine an occasion on which your own intake of fluid has gone up or down. This could be a social evening, when you had several drinks, or it could be a time when you were unable to obtain a drink, even though you were very thirsty.

Describe, in a short sentence, the situation you have imagined and the effect it had on your output of fluid.

Commentary

Here is an answer provided by a nurse who tried this activity:

'I can remember a skiing holiday when I spent all day up a mountain and only had a cup of coffee at lunch time. I was struck afterwards by the fact that I hadn't needed to go to the lavatory all day.'

This person must have been losing a lot of water by sweating and evaporation in the dry air and sunshine. She drank very little and therefore replaced very little fluid. Her blood plasma would contain a reduced amount of water. In response, her output of urine was greatly reduced. In this way, the amount of water in her internal environment was kept constant.

The opposite to this situation is the increase in output which we observe after an increased intake. In both cases we see examples of the way the body automatically adjusts its internal environment, a process known as **homeostasis**. This is the most important concept in physiology and you will be returning to it many times in this unit. It is through homeostasis that the cells from which our bodies are made can continue to function. An understanding of the concept helps nurses to appreciate the importance of the internal environment, both in healthy human tissue and in areas where healing is taking place.

The adjustments which you have just considered happen without any conscious effort. The body recognises that an internal change has occurred and some regulatory action takes place. All homeostatic processes occur in this way. In the case of fluid regulation, the recognition is done by specialised parts of the nervous system called **osmoreceptors**. These detect changes in the amount of water and dissolved substances in the plasma and cause nerve signals to be sent to a part of the brain which regulates the amount of a chemical messenger **(hormone)** in the bloodstream. The hormone causes the kidneys to produce more or less urine. We will look at this process in more detail in Session Two.

Coping with change

Deprivation of water is much more serious than deprivation of food, and its effects provide a useful illustration of the way in which the body copes with change. To assist our understanding of these effects we will first consider a problem that many people experience at some time in their lives.

ACTIVITY 4

Think about an occasion where you have been out in the hot sun for several hours and have felt unwell as a result. If you have not had the experience yourself, consider another person who has. Briefly describe the effects produced by this exposure.

Commentary

The effects of too much sunshine can be unpleasant. You may have been affected slightly or you may have suffered more severe heatstroke. You might have experienced some or all of the following:

- headache
- thirst
- nausea
- vomiting
- sunburn
- fainting.

In very severe reactions people experience confusion and even unconsciousness.

These symptoms are due to loss of fluid from the body, caused by the heat. The reduction in fluid volume is detected by the osmoreceptors and a hormone is sent to the kidneys, slowing down or stopping the production of urine and thus conserving water in the body. This is vital to ensure that the environment of the cells is kept constant, but it incurs a cost. As the urine output is reduced, so is the removal of waste products from the blood. These build up in the bloodstream and produce the unpleasant effects just described.

These effects occur when water intake and output are out of balance. When fluid is lost more rapidly than it is gained a person becomes dehydrated. This results from illness, as well as from heat exposure.

ACTIVITY 5

We would now like you to consider the causes and effects of dehydration. You may have encountered a person who is dehydrated in hospital or in other situations. If not, please take the opportunity to talk to someone who knows about the condition – a nursing colleague, for example.

1 Identify at least one cause of dehydration in people receiving health care.

2 Write a short description of the appearance of a dehydrated person.

Commentary

1 You may have identified one or more of the following:

- raised temperature and sweating
- nausea and vomiting
- diarrhoea
- unwillingness or inability to take fluids, for a variety of reasons.

2 A dehydrated person may have:

- dry mouth, dry tongue and sore, cracked lips
- loss of skin elasticity (If you pinch the skin on the back of someone's hand it normally springs back into place – if the person is dehydrated the skin fold takes much longer to move back to normal.)
- sunken eyes
- lethargy
- rapid weak pulse
- very reduced urine output
- dark, concentrated urine.

All of these are the effects of a reduction in the volume of body fluids.

Patients who have been sweating or suffering from diarrhoea and vomiting are not only short of water. They also lose some of the dissolved substances from their body fluids, so that the balance between them becomes upset. To bring the balance back to normal they need both water and salt. This is the basis of the emergency treatment of ill children, where a rehydration mixture containing glucose and salts in water is given. Water alone is not enough.

2: Fluids in the wrong places

We hope that you now have an outline in your mind of the body fluids and the way that their volumes are controlled. Now we can take a closer look at the problem of misplaced fluid.

The problem of oedema

ACTIVITY 6   ALLOW 5 MINUTES

This activity is based on the first of our case studies. These are all based on real people that we have cared for, and you are likely to come across similar people yourselves. Please read through the case study and then consider the question at the end. The story begins about six years ago.

Mr Granville was first admitted to a medical ward at this time. His home was in the countryside, about 40 miles from hospital, and he got few visitors. Perhaps because of this, he was very quiet and subdued. He spent long periods during the day sitting in the day room and was not very keen about moving from his favourite chair.

When taken back to bed for a rest after lunch his slippers were difficult to remove and they left an impression on his feet, which were very swollen, with tight, shiny skin.

When the nurse taking care of Mr Granville noticed this he tested the swelling by pressing firmly with his finger. The swelling was firm and the finger left a depression which lasted for some time.

Assuming that the swelling in Mr Granville's feet is caused by fluid, can you suggest reasons for the observations described in the case study? Please note your ideas in the space below.

Commentary

Your reasons could have been something like this. For some reason, Mr Granville's body contained excess fluid which found its way, when he was sitting down, into the lowest parts of his body, his legs and feet. The fluid accumulated in the tissues under his skin, causing the skin to stretch, and thus become smooth and shiny. The waterlogged tissues were firm, but it was easy to displace the fluid by steady pressure, leaving a depression which was slow to fill out again.

As we explained at the beginning of this session, an accumulation of fluid in the wrong place, such as this, is termed oedema. There are a number of different types of oedema, arising in different ways. In this instance we have observed **pitting oedema**, so called because the tissue retains the marks of pressure applied.

This kind of oedema can easily be observed, because its effects are directly visible. It is caused by an increase in the volume of intercellular fluid in the surface tissues. However, unwanted fluids can accumulate in the internal organs as well, resulting, for example, in oedema of the tissues of the brain, the digestive system and the lungs.

ACTIVITY 7 ALLOW 5 MINUTES

For each of the three examples in the previous paragraph, can you imagine the effect that the oedema would have on the affected person? For example, consider what effect excess fluid in the tissues of the brain is likely to have, bearing in mind that the brain is enclosed in the bony skull. Even if you have done no physiology at all before starting this unit, try to reason out your answers to this question.

Commentary

Fluid in and around the brain tissue will produce swelling and pressure. This will result in headache. Indeed, one type of migraine headache is caused by oedema of a small area of tissue behind the forehead – demonstrating how severe the effect can be.

Accumulation of fluid in and around the digestive organs will result in abdominal swelling and pressure on the stomach and other parts of the digestive system. This will produce a feeling of fullness and therefore loss of appetite. If it gets worse, nausea and vomiting may follow.

Fluid in the lungs – **pulmonary oedema** – will interfere with the process of breathing, producing coughing and breathlessness.

ACTIVITY 8
ALLOW **10** MINUTES

Let's return to the case study of Mr Granville again and provide some more information about him. Before answering the question that follows this part of the case study, perhaps you could discuss his nursing care with a colleague, preferably someone with experience of caring for people like him.

Mr Granville was admitted to hospital because he had had a fall at home and a slight stroke was suspected. He was then aged 73 and had been treated by his GP for 'heart trouble' for the past ten years.

One week after admission his condition was reassessed and it was decided that he could be discharged to a rehabilitation ward. The objective of rehabilitation would be to help him become mobile again, so that he could return home to his familiar surroundings.

What problems will the oedema we have observed cause for Mr Granville's rehabilitation? Please consider this question, and note down your ideas in the space below.

Commentary

It is going to be difficult to get Mr Granville walking again if he cannot wear good footwear and if his feet are uncomfortable or painful.

His skin is under pressure from the underlying fluid and may easily become damaged, causing an ulcer. He is therefore at some risk. The oedema is a potential cause of problems, which may delay his return home.

So you can see that oedema can be a serious matter for a patient and needs to be well managed if its effects are to be minimised.

How oedema is produced

Let's now consider the cause of Mr Granville's oedema. It has arisen because the amount of fluid going into the tissues is greater than the amount leaving them – so again we see the effect of a dynamic system getting out of balance. But before going into more detail about the process involved you need to take a look at the system which carries blood around the body.

The blood vessels bringing blood from the heart (the **arteries**) divide up into smaller vessels (**arterioles**) and finally into very small **capillaries**. These run in between the tissue cells, forming the **capillary network**. They then join up again to form the vessels carrying blood back to the heart (**veins**). The walls of these capillaries separate the plasma from the intercellular fluid. There is an exchange of substances between these two, but normally the amount of fluid in each remains constant. This happens because the forces pushing fluid in and out of the plasma are balanced and so the overall result is 'no change'. The two forces are **hydrostatic** pressure, which pushes fluid out, and **osmotic** pressure, which draws water back into the plasma.

Hydrostatic pressure is, in effect, the same as the **blood pressure** inside the blood vessels. This is the pressure of the blood in the vessels, resulting from the force generated by the heart and the resistance of the blood vessel walls. As the heart contracts, blood is forced through the arteries. Their walls can stretch to a certain degree because they contain elastic material, but the surge of blood is resisted by the wall. (From now on 'blood pressure' will be abbreviated to BP.)

As you will see in Session Three, the heart beat causes blood to surge through the vessels in regular waves. The BP is highest as a wave passes a particular point and falls to its lowest value between waves. So measurements of BP always contain two figures – one for the highest value and one for the lowest. Please bear this in mind in the discussion that follows.

The capillaries have very thin walls. By the time the blood gets to these tiny vessels its pressure is much reduced and the waves have levelled out, but there is still sufficient hydrostatic pressure to force water and small dissolved molecules out of the plasma to form the intercellular fluid.

After dividing among the tissue cells, capillaries rejoin to form veins carrying blood back to the heart. But how does the fluid get back into these capillaries? It is easy to imagine fluid being forced out of tiny blood vessels by the residual force of the pumping heart, but less easy to imagine how it gets back in. Yet it must normally get back in: otherwise we would all be subject to severe oedema. The answer is that water is 'pulled' back into the plasma by **osmosis** (the result of the *osmotic* pressure that we noted above).

Osmosis is the term used to describe the movement of water from one location to another across a **semi-permeable** membrane – that is, a thin barrier which allows water but not dissolved substances to cross. The outer layer of any cell is a **cell membrane**. These are very complex structures, performing a variety of functions. However, since they do act as membranes of the kind we are describing by allowing water to cross and holding some dissolved substances back, we can think of them in rather simplified terms for the purposes of this discussion.

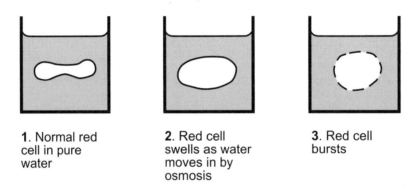

1. Normal red cell in pure water

2. Red cell swells as water moves in by osmosis

3. Red cell bursts

Figure 2 The effect of osmotic pressure on a red blood cell

Red blood cells are each surrounded by a membrane. *Figure 2* shows three diagrams of a red blood cell in a container of water. In the first the cell is its normal disc shape. It contains a large amount of protein, especially **haemoglobin**, the protein responsible for the transport of oxygen. This makes the environment inside the red cell more concentrated than pure water. The interior of the cell therefore has a higher osmotic pressure than the fluid outside.

The result is that water is drawn into the cell. If the membrane was very elastic, water would continue to enter until the osmotic pressure inside the cell became the same as that outside. In reality the red cell can only expand to a certain point; then it bursts.

This is why when patients are given fluid directly into the circulation (intravenously) a solution containing glucose and salts, rather than pure water, is always used. Pure water would reduce the osmotic pressure of the plasma, causing water to enter the red cells.

Figure 2 demonstrates how water always moves from a dilute solution to a more concentrated one, when the two are separated by a membrane which allows the water but not the dissolved substances (such as salts and proteins) to pass across.

We have discussed what happens to a cell in water. The opposite situation is also of physiological importance. When cells are in contact with fluids that are more highly concentrated than their contents the same osmotic process takes place, but with a different result. Water moves from the less to the more concentrated fluid. It therefore moves out of the cells and into the fluid surrounding them, across the cell membrane. This movement continues until the osmotic pressure on both sides of the membrane is equal. The cells lose water and may become shrunken and shrivelled.

The osmotic pressure in the plasma is produced by the plasma proteins. There are more proteins in the plasma than in the intercellular fluid, so its osmotic pressure is higher. This tends to draw water back into the capillaries unless opposed by hydrostatic pressure.

So in all parts of the capillary network, we have two forces, hydrostatic pressure (H) and osmotic pressure (O), acting on the fluid in the capillaries. Where H is greater than O, fluid leaves the plasma. Where O is greater than H, it flows the other way.

Some people find the idea of osmotic pressure 'pulling' water into a strong solution a little confusing. We are used to thinking of pressure in terms of 'pushing'. Perhaps it is better to think of the pressures acting in the blood system as forces applied to fluids, which cause them to move in various directions. So osmotic pressure is a force which drives water from a weaker solution into a stronger one and hydrostatic pressure is a force caused by fluid being 'squeezed' inside a tube. It acts against the walls of the tube and tends to drive water out of the tube at any point where it can escape.

Measuring these forces often has to be done indirectly. The strength of any force can be determined by the strength of the force needed to overcome it. This is what the 'old fashioned' method of measuring BP, using a **sphygmomanometer**, does. A force is applied over a blood vessel by means of an inflated cuff and increased until it stops the blood flowing. It is then gradually lowered until the blood just begins to flow again. When that starts to happen, we know that the strength of the force driving the blood is greater than the force which has been applied. This gives a measure of the highest BP value.

The sphygmomanometer cuff is attached to a glass column containing mercury. The force in the cuff as it is inflated is measured by the height to which the mercury column is raised. That height is recorded as millimetres (mm). The pressure of blood and the other forces operating in the system is therefore recorded in millimetres of mercury (mmHg – Hg being the chemical symbol for mercury).

The use of these units for pressure measurement goes back a long way. It originates from the study of the earth's atmosphere. This is a mass of gases which rests on the earth and exerts a force upon its surface. The pressure of the atmosphere is the amount of force exerted on a given area. This was originally measured with a barometer, which records pressures as the height of a column of mercury which the atmosphere pressure can support. From this the sphygmomanometer developed, and physiological pressures were recorded in units of mmHg.

In recent years scientists have standardised measurement procedures so that everything may be measured in terms of three units – kilograms (kg), metres (m) and seconds (s). This is the **SI (Système International)** system. Under this system, pressure is measured as force per unit area, and the name for the unit of measurement is the pascal (**Pa**). A thousand pascals is a kilopascal (**kPa**). You may see physiological pressures expressed as **Pa** or **kPa**, rather than the older term of mmHg. The relationship between them is :

1kPa = 7.5mmHg. We will use the older term in this unit, as it is still in very general use.

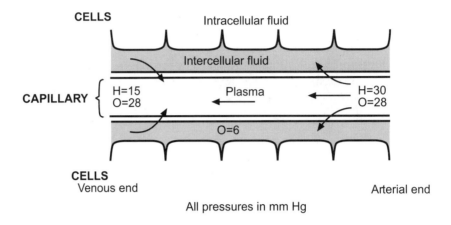

Figure 3 Pressures in the capillary networks

ACTIVITY 9   ALLOW 5 MINUTES

Figure 3 shows the pressures in part of the capillary network. After studying the diagram, write a sentence to summarise what happens at the arterial end (where blood arrives in the tissues) and another summarising what happens at the venous end (where blood leaves the tissues).

Commentary

Your summary will probably be along these lines:

The hydrostatic pressure drops as the blood flows from the arterial to the venous end of the capillary networks.

At the arterial end the combined pressures (or forces) moving fluid out of the capillary are higher than those in the other direction.

At the venous end the reverse is true.

Let's look at the actual figures. First, at the arterial end, the force moving fluid out is the sum of H in the capillary and O in the intercellular fluid – that is 30 + 6mmHg. The force moving fluid the other way – back into the capillary – is due solely to the osmotic pressure in the capillary. There is no H in the intercellular fluid. Therefore we have:

Force moving fluid *out* of capillary = H (capillary) + O (intercellular fluid)
= 30 + 6 = 36

Force moving fluid *into* the capillary = O (capillary) = 28

The difference between these = 36 − 28 = 8 mmHg

This is the *total* force moving fluid out at the arterial end.

Now let's consider the venous end of the capillary network.

Here:

Force moving fluid *out* of capillary = H (capillary) + O (intercellular fluid)
= 15 + 6 = 21

Force moving fluid into capillary = O (capillary)
= 28

The difference between these = 28 − 21 = 7 mmHg
This is the *total* force driving fluid back into the capillaries at the venous end.

Pressures in the capillary network vary in different tissues, but the important factor, in terms of the volume of intercellular fluid, is the difference between the arterial and venous ends. Whatever the actual pressures may be, if the two sets of forces are balanced the volume of this fluid is normal because the amount of fluid leaving the plasma is the same as the amount returning. However, if the balance between H and O changes at either end, then more fluid may be forced out than returns – resulting in the occurrence of oedema.

The analogy of a pond can be used to illustrate this idea further. Imagine this as an artificial garden pond, fed by a natural stream. If it rains heavily, the stream flowing in will run faster than the outlet stream. The pond will overflow and the garden becomes waterlogged. The same thing will happen if the outlet stream is blocked with fallen leaves.

In the case of the formation of intercellular fluid we are considering a rather more complex situation in which the inflows and outflows are each the result of the balance between two opposing forces. But the principle is just the same. If you think about each of these forces you should be able to work out what effects any change will have on the volume of intercellular fluid – in other words, what contribution it will make to the development of oedema. The next two activities provide an opportunity to do this and to consolidate your work in this session.

ACTIVITY 10 · ALLOW 3 MINUTES

You may need a little longer to review Session One.

Here is a picture of a child who is very ill because he lives in a part of the world severely affected by famine. He has suffered from a shortage of protein for a long time.

After observing the physical appearance of this little boy, please describe the extent of any oedema you can see and, using the information gained in Session One of this unit, suggest why it has occurred.

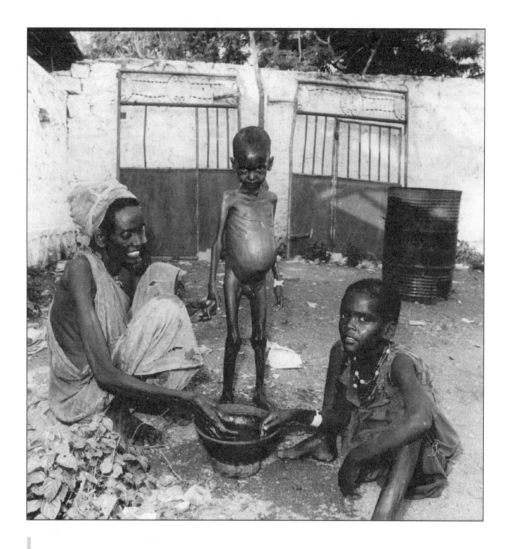

Commentary

The things that are most noticeable about this child are his very thin limbs and swollen abdomen and legs. The swelling is caused by oedema. In this case the oedema is due to the reduced osmotic pressure of the plasma. The prolonged shortage of dietary proteins has reduced the concentration of plasma proteins which, as you noted earlier, are largely responsible for the osmotic pressure of the plasma. There is therefore less force driving water back into the plasma from the cellular fluid, and so it accumulates, particularly in the lower parts of the body, such as the legs and abdomen.

Now let's review the effects of the other force – the hydrostatic pressure, which forces fluid out of the arterial capillaries or prevents it getting back into the venous capillaries.

ACTIVITY 11   ALLOW 3 MINUTES

Here is some more information from Mr Granville's case study. Please consider it and then answer the questions.

When Mr Granville was admitted to the medical ward on the occasion described in Activity 6 his notes recorded that he had been treated by his family doctor for raised BP and had previously suffered a mild heart attack. Amongst the medication he brought with him were what he called his 'water tablets', which his GP prescribed regularly.

1   Thinking about this aspect of his condition and ideas of balance in the capillary network, what effect might his failing heart have on the volume of his intercellular fluid? Record your answer in the space below:

2   How do you think 'water tablets' might help to relieve Mr Granville's symptoms?

Commentary

1   The result of Mr Granville's heart attack was, probably, some damage to his heart muscle, reducing its ability to pump blood right round his body as effectively as before. If this occurred, blood might stagnate in the lowest parts of his body, his legs and his feet, because there was insufficient force to drive blood from there back up to his heart.

The accumulation of blood at the venous end of the capillary network would increase the hydrostatic pressure there. This would then be greater than the osmotic pressure in the plasma and so more fluid would leave the plasma than was drawn back.

2   Clearly, some of Mr Granville's problems are caused by an excess of fluid. This can be seen as oedema in his legs, but it might also affect major organs in his body, such as his lungs. Removing excess fluid will help. 'Water tablets' are drugs which increase the output of urine and therefore help to remove excess fluid.

This overview of the formation of intercellular fluid has, inevitably, simplified a very complex process. For example, we have not mentioned the formation of **lymph**. This results from a mechanism by which small volumes of protein-containing fluid which are extruded from the capillaries, play an important protective and transport role, and are then collected for return to the blood through a system of lymphatic vessels. The volumes of lymph produced are small in relation to the total volume of intercellular fluid in any part of the capillary network, and we have therefore disregarded them in this session, where we have been discussing the blood circulation. However, there are conditions in which the lymph drainage vessels are damaged and lymph accumulates in one part of the body. This can occur, for example, after surgery for breast cancer when part of the drainage system in the armpit is involved in the procedure. Lymph may accumulate in the affected arm, which becomes very swollen. This condition is termed **lymphoedema.**

Caring for a person with peripheral oedema

We have discussed the way in which oedema in the tissues in the lower parts of the body is caused. This type of oedema is called **peripheral oedema,** referring to the fact that the oedema occurs at the parts of the body furthest away from the centre. The next activity asks you to consider how nurses can support people with this problem.

Or a little longer if you plan to discuss this with a colleague

ACTIVITY 12   ALLOW **10** MINUTES

Mr Granville needed skilled nursing care to ensure that his peripheral oedema was well managed and interfered as little as possible with his rehabilitation.

Consider his case, using the information provided so far. Either working on your own, or after discussion with colleagues, list some of the nursing actions which might have been included in his care plan.

Commentary

Here are some suggestions that you might have made, with some added information to explain them:

Reduce the amount of time Mr Granville spends sitting in a chair. When he is sitting down encourage him to raise his legs on a stool to improve the venous blood flow and reduce the effects of gravity on the fluid in his feet.

Encourage gentle exercise. Muscle activity improves the venous circulation.

Advise Mr Granville to take care of his skin, particularly on his legs and feet. Any small scratch over an oedematous area will allow intercellular fluid to leak onto the surface, producing a risk of infection. Because of the extra fluid in such an area the blood supply to the surface tissues will be hindered. Therefore healing of any small wound will be slower than normal because healing processes require a good blood supply.

Tight shoes and socks (particularly socks with elasticated tops) should be avoided, as they will further increase the pressure in the lower leg veins.

Carry out accurate recording of fluid intake and output to check fluid balance and to assess the effectiveness of his treatment and care.

A more accurate way of assessing changes in the volume of the oedema is to weigh Mr Granville every day. To be effective this must be carried out at the same time each day and in the same way.

I hope that this discussion has shown how unbalanced forces lead to an accumulation of fluid which settles to the lowest possible place under the influence of gravity and how nursing care can help to minimise the effects. An understanding of the physiological process underlying the production of peripheral oedema improves the nurse's ability to plan and evaluate care.

Summary of Session One

- All body fluids are based on water.

- The fluid in the body is found mainly in the cells (intracellular fluid), surrounding the cells (intercellular fluid) and in the plasma.

- The composition of the intercellular fluid provides a stable environment for the survival of living cells.

- The maintenance of that environment is termed homeostastis.

- The volume of water and the concentration of dissolved substances are critical features of that environment.

- Homeostatic mechanisms exist to keep these features constant, despite fluctuating inputs and outputs.

- The intercellular fluid is in a dynamic state. Its volume is controlled by the balance of forces in the capillary network.

- If these forces are unbalanced dehydration or oedema will result.

- Oedema can occur in most parts of the body, such as the brain and lungs. In the surface tissues it is readily visible as peripheral oedema.

- Peripheral oedema interferes with mobility and puts the skin at risk. Nursing has an important role in its management.

Please check through the summary points and make sure that they are all clear to you before moving on to Session Two.

There are many causes of oedema. You have touched on some of them as you studied Mr Granville's case. In Session Two you will look at the way oedema can arise when problems occur in the body's system for regulating the amount of water and dissolved substances in the body fluids.

SESSION TWO

Regulatory problems

Introduction

Session One was all about water and the results of imbalances in the amount of water leaving and passing back into the capillaries. However, body fluids do not consist only of water. They contain many kinds of dissolved substances. The levels of these substances in and around the cells are kept constant, thus providing the internal environment which the living cells need.

The concentration of dissolved substances in the body fluids is controlled by the renal system, which consists of the kidneys and associated structures. The kidneys are responsible for removing unwanted dissolved substances and excess water from the body. They adjust the amounts of these substances in the urine in a way that keeps the body fluids constant, despite great variation in the inputs to the body. This **regulatory process** has far-reaching effects, one being the control of the amount of water leaving and re-entering the plasma. So, as we discuss the action of the kidneys we will also be able to consider another way in which oedema occurs.

Session objectives

When you have completed this session you should be able to:

- outline the structure of the normal kidney and the way in which urine is produced
- explain the effects of reduced fluid intake
- explain why fluids are given, as a matter of urgency, to casualties who have suffered blood loss
- describe the role of the kidney in the homeostatic processes which regulate BP
- explain the principle of feedback control as it applies to the renin/angiotensin system
- describe and explain the symptoms of chronic and acute renal failure
- discuss the role of the clinical nurse specialist working in a renal unit
- outline the relationship between renal and cardiac function.

1: Chronic renal failure

The activity that follows asks you to think about a person whose kidney function is of great concern to all his carers.

ACTIVITY 13   ALLOW 15 MINUTES

Caring for a person with renal failure

Please read Resource 1, the story of Michael. Then consider the following question:

What symptoms did Michael show as his renal failure started to affect him? Make a list of the symptoms he experienced before being admitted to hospital for the first time.

Commentary

Your list will have included some or all of the following, which are described in Resource 1:

- nausea
- tiredness
- feeling generally unwell
- vomiting
- breathlessness
- headaches
- deterioration of the sense of taste
- deteriorating eyesight
- raised BP (hypertension).

All these unpleasant things are caused by disturbances resulting from failure of the regulatory mechanism of kidneys. After completing this session you will be able to explain why each of them occurs. First, let's take a look at the very important structures which carry out this vital activity – the kidneys.

2: Healthy kidneys

What the kidneys do

In adults the kidneys are 10–12 cm long and 5–7.5 cm wide. Each weighs about 150 g. As you build up a picture of the amount of work that they do you may be impressed that such relatively small organs can do so much.

Figure 4 shows where the kidneys are located and their blood supply. Notice that they are directly connected to the major artery and vein in the abdomen. The vessel bringing blood into the kidney (the renal artery) is large, indicating that a lot of blood flows into the kidney each time the heart beats.

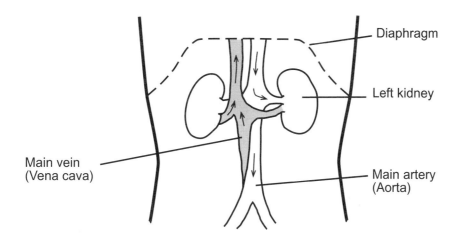

Figure 4 The relationship of the kidneys to the major blood vessels

During the course of 24 hours, the volume of blood flowing through the kidneys is 1700 litres. Since the total volume of plasma in an adult is approximately three litres it is clear that all the blood in the circulation must pass through the kidneys many times each day.

The blood which passes through the kidneys is sometimes diluted by extra fluid intake and sometimes more concentrated by either fluid loss or extra intake of dissolved substances. The job of the kidneys is to adjust the concentration of the blood, moment by moment, as it passes through. It does this by removing water and dissolved substances as necessary to adjust the concentration. *Figure 5* summarises this function.

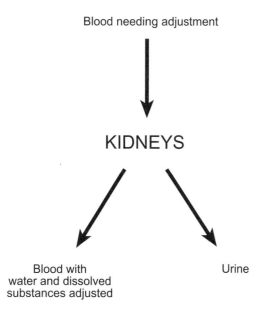

Figure 5 Inputs and outputs of the kidney

As if this wasn't enough, the kidneys carry out several other tasks as well. For example, they:

- remove harmful substances from the blood
- produce a hormone which helps maintain an adequate BP
- produce a hormone which is essential for the formation of new red blood cells in the bone marrow.

In order to understand how the kidneys perform these functions we need to consider their internal structure.

ACTIVITY 14　　　　　ALLOW 10 MINUTES

Lambs' kidneys are very similar to those of humans. You might find it helpful to obtain one from the butcher and have a close look at it in the raw state.

- Describe how the whole kidney looks first.
- Then cut it in half lengthways and describe the appearance of the cut section.
- Finally, see if you can explain what you observe, as far as possible.

Commentary

Did you notice that the whole kidney was:

- soft and spongy?
- deep red in colour?
- surrounded by a tough 'envelope' of tissue?

When you cut it in half you would probably notice two distinct areas of colour – deep red round the outside and paler towards the centre.

The kidney is full of blood. In life, blood is being pumped through it each time the heart beats. After death the soft tissue still retains blood, although it is much less full, of course. The kidney tissue is very delicate and the surrounding tissue protects it. (Did you notice how difficult it was to make a hole in this envelope?)

Unless you have studied the anatomy of the kidney before, you will not have been able to explain its internal appearance. This is what we will consider next.

The idea of the kidney as a simple filter is much too crude. Blood must pass through it in a very controlled way if its composition is to be precisely adjusted. But we have already noted that the kidney deals with very large volumes of blood. In order to do this it is not just one filter – it is composed of millions of separate filters, each one of which can be regulated to get the result required.

The separate filters are coiled tubes termed **nephrons**. Each one opens into a duct where the urine collects at one end and has a cup-shaped structure (the **glomerular capsule**) at the other. The renal artery divides up into smaller and smaller branches in the kidney. Each branch forms a knot of capillaries (the **glomerulus**) which fits into the glomerular capsule. Fluid is forced out of these capillaries by hydrostatic pressure in the way described in Session One.

ACTIVITY 15

ALLOW **10** MINUTES

Or more if you need to review Session One

If necessary, check back to Session One and revise the forces which cause fluid to move out of the capillaries, in the capillary network, to form the intercellular fluid. Then look at *Figure 6*, which shows the knot of capillaries bringing blood to a nephron. The forces influencing the movement of fluid out of these capillaries are shown by arrows, each of which has a number on it to show its strength. We would like you to:

● Label these arrows to show what forces they represent

● Use the numbers on the arrows to calculate the strength of the force which pushes fluid out of the glomerulus in the normal kidney.

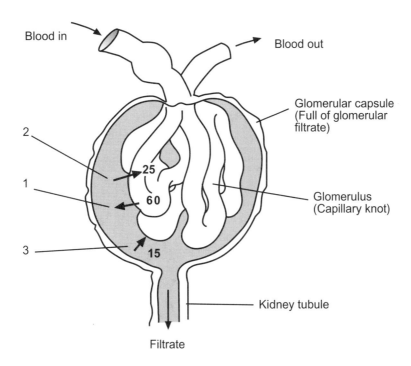

Figure 6 The Glomerular capsule
(section through to show forces acting to form glomerular filtrate)

Commentary

There are three forces working together here. The largest is the hydrostatic pressure in the capillary (60 mmHg) forcing fluid out (Arrow 1). This is counteracted by the osmotic pressure of the plasma (25 mmHg) drawing fluid back in (Arrow 2). There is also the hydrostatic pressure of the fluid in the glomerular capsule, opposing the passage of fluid out of the plasma (15mmHg) (Arrow 3). This fluid has no protein so its osmotic pressure is very low. We can call it zero. So the actual force pushing fluid out is:

60 − (25 + 15) = 20 mmHg

This is the force which pushes fluid out of the glomerulus into the top of the nephron.

The walls of the capillaries are very thin – the thickness of a single flat cell. Water and small molecules can pass across these thin walls under pressures such as the one you have just calculated. Large molecules such as proteins, however, do not pass across at low pressures. If, for any reason, the hydrostatic pressure in the glomerulus becomes very high, proteins will be forced out of the plasma and will appear in the urine.

Under normal circumstances, then, the fluid which is forced out of the knot of capillaries (the **glomerular filtrate**) has the same composition as the plasma, except for the proteins, which remain behind. It contains many substances, all of them important, and the job of the kidney is to put back into the blood the amounts of those substances needed to regulate its composition. Remember that this blood plasma is then going to circulate around the body and will give rise to the intercellular fluid, as described in Session One.

Substances regulated by the kidney

In this introductory course there is not enough space to discuss all the dissolved substances which are regulated by the kidney. We will concentrate on three of them – salt, glucose and urea.

The plasma contains several substances that are termed 'salts'. We are going to discuss the most common of these, from which the group gets its name, common salt, which we will simply call 'salt'. Salt enters the blood plasma directly from food passing through the digestive system. It takes part in many important activities, including the transmission of nerve impulses. Salt, in its solid form, consists of **molecules** of **sodium chloride**. When it dissolves in water the molecules come apart – speaking scientifically we should say that they dissociate into particles – each of which carries a very small electrical charge. These charged particles are **ions** of sodium (which has a positive charge) and chlorine (which has a negative charge). In the solid state salt these opposite charges hold the particles together in a stable structure. Substances which dissociate in this way conduct electricity when in solution. They are termed **electrolytes**. All the substances commonly called salts are electrolytes. The concentration of salt and other electrolytes in the intercellular fluid is vital for the well-being of the cells.

Glucose also enters the plasma from the diet. It is the main product of the digestion of food and forms the principal energy source for all the cells of the body. If the concentration of glucose in the blood is too high or too low, problems arise.

ACTIVITY 16: OPTIONAL   ALLOW 10 MINUTES

If you have studied the Biochemistry unit you might like to revise the role of glucose at this point. The relevant section of this unit is provided as Resource 2. It is not essential to do this, but you may find it helpful as background reading.

Urea is formed from the digestion and breakdown of proteins. It is a waste product and needs to be removed from the body. The concentration of urea in the plasma is not problematic until it exceeds a certain level, when the symptoms of **uraemia** become evident. A person who is becoming uraemic loses his or her appetite, becomes nauseated, and has an unpleasant taste in the mouth. As urea levels in the blood increase other unpleasant symptoms develop such as vomiting, skin irritation and muscle cramps. The person may seem irritable and confused, eventually progressing from drowsiness to unconsciousness. If untreated, the condition is fatal.

How the kidney deals with dissolved substances

We will now consider how the kidney deals with water and these three dissolved materials. When the blood reaches the top of the nephron the glomerular filtrate is forced out into the capsule. The filtrate has the same composition as the plasma, except for the proteins. Suppose, for example, that a person has just eaten a packet of crisps. The salt will be quickly absorbed into his blood and the plasma will have a higher salt concentration than normal. So will the fluid entering the nephron. The nephron's task is to get rid of that excess salt and return the blood plasma concentrate to normal.

Now the kidney is not able simply to pull the excess salt out from the plasma as the blood flows through the kidney. In theory it could do this, but it would require an enormous amount of energy to deal with salt and all the other things it has to extract. What it actually does is to take fluid out of the plasma, adjust its concentration and put it back in the blood, allowing everything that is unwanted to flow on as urine. It does this in a very efficient way, expending the minimum possible energy. Even so, the kidneys need as much energy as the heart beating at its resting rate.

This complex set of events is made possible by the structure of the nephron itself. There are three distinct regions, as *Figure 7a* shows.

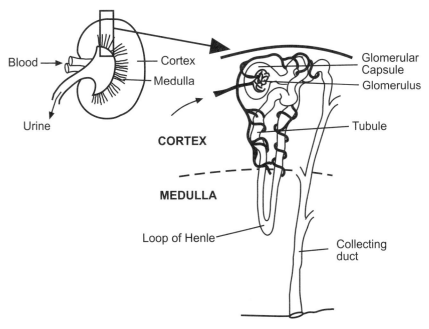

Figure 7a The structure of the nephron

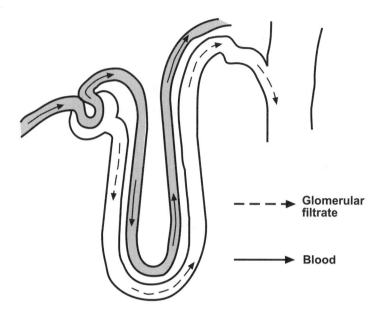

Figure 7b Diagrammatic structure of the nephron to show blood supply

This diagram shows a single nephron. The capillaries surrounding it have been simplified. In the living kidney, the whole nephron is wrapped in a network of capillaries which are taking blood back into the veins. In other words, they are carrying the blood from which fluid has been forced out at the top of the nephron. So this blood is, in effect, flowing back alongside the nephron. *Figure 7b* simplifies the structure further by depicting both the nephron tubule and the blood supply as single, straight tubes in order to show the relationship between them.

In the first part of the nephron, the tube is very 'leaky', and allows glucose, salt and most of the water to be taken back into the blood in the capillary.

In the second part, the loop of Henle – the 'hairpin' structure – allows the fluid flowing down to be concentrated at the bottom of the loop, by adjusting the amounts of salt and water being taken back into the capillaries. This structure occurs only in animals which are capable of producing concentrated urine (i.e. birds and mammals, including humans). Several drugs used to promote the flow of urine (**diuretics**) act on this region of the nephron. The 'water tablets' which Mr Granville was taking are diuretics.

In the final section of the nephron fine adjustments are made to the concentration of the urine, which then flows into the collecting duct.

The result of these processes is that the urine has a very different concentration of salts and other substances to the plasma.

ACTIVITY 17   ALLOW 5 MINUTES

Table 4 shows the relative concentrations of some of the substances which enter and leave the nephrons in 24 hours.

	Glomerular filtrate	Urine
Water	170 litres	1.5 litres
Glucose	170 g	none
Salt	1180 g	14 g
Urea	51 g	30 g

Table 4 Composition of glomerular filtrate and urine over 24 hours in a healthy adult

> After considering this table, see if you can summarise the events which occur as the filtrate passes along the nephrons. Describe these events in your own words in the space below.

Commentary

Your description might have been along these lines. Comparing the fluid that is forced out of the plasma in 24 hours with the urine which actually leaves the body it is clear that:

- most of the water is taken back (reabsorbed)
- all of the glucose is reabsorbed
- most of the salt is reabsorbed
- about 60% of the urea is removed in the urine.

In this way, the composition of the plasma is kept constant, because the substances which are taken back are those that are needed for this purpose.

The figures in *Table 4* show how much of each substance is forced out of the plasma in a 24-hour period. During that time, of course, the composition of the plasma will vary according to what a person has been doing. After eating a heavy meal the concentration of glucose goes up, while after working hard in hot weather the amount of water and salt goes down, as a result of excessive sweating. The composition of the plasma changes from moment to moment and the job of the kidney is to respond to these changes by varying the amounts of water, salt, glucose and urea which are taken back into the plasma from the glomerular filtrate.

This variation is brought about by a control system which acts on several parts of the nephron to influence reabsorption. One element of this system is the hormone ADH (**antidiuretic hormone**). The effect of this hormone is to increase the rate of reabsorption of water in the nephron, causing water to return to the capillaries. The amount of this hormone circulating in the blood and reaching the kidneys rises and falls according to the composition of the plasma.

ACTIVITY 18   ALLOW 3 MINUTES

1 Review the last section and, based on the information which it contains, write a sentence to describe what will happen when the ADH level falls.

2 Based on your answer to the first question, can you guess what will happen to the level of ADH in the plasma if you drink a large volume of water?

Commentary

Here is one way in which you might have described some of the changes in ADH levels which can occur.

1 If the level of ADH falls for any reason, less water will be reabsorbed by the nephrons and so more urine will be produced.

2 Your answer here will be something of a guess (unless you have studied this topic before), but it will be an informed guess, based on what you are learning about homeostasis. If you drink a lot of water, the amount of water in your plasma will increase. In order to bring it back to normal, the body must remove the excess fluid. It can do this by decreasing the level of ADH and thus having the effect which I have already described. A sentence to sum this up could be along these lines:

'Because of the increased amount of water in the plasma, the level of ADH falls, less water is reabsorbed from the glomerular filtrate and more urine is produced.'

Intake and output of fluid

In Activity 4 you considered your own experience of the effect of water shortage and in Activity 5 you looked at dehydration, which occurs in people whose water balance is seriously disturbed by input not matching output over a period of time. Both these activities referred to thirst.

Thirst

The natural response to a lack of water is the sensation that we call 'thirst'. This is a very powerful and unpleasant sensation which, when severe, leads to a strong drive to obtain water. It is caused by a combination of two things. First, osmoreceptors in the brain detect changes in the concentration of the plasma. Secondly, receptors of a different type in the chest detect how full the main blood vessels are. If the total volume of plasma in the body is low there will be less volume in the blood vessels and they will not be stretched so much as the blood passes through. Both these kinds of receptors stimulate the brain to produce the conscious sensation of thirst. They also stimulate production of more ADH, cutting down the loss of fluid.

It is known that when people are thirsty they will drink a large volume of fluid very rapidly, but only sufficient to replace what has been lost. Astronauts in space tend not to drink as much as they should. They do not feel as thirsty as usual, even when short of water, probably because, in the absence of gravity, the volume of blood in the vessels in the chest is higher, since blood is not held down in the legs and feet.

Passing urine

Micturition is the technical word for the action of passing urine. In young babies this is a reflex action – i.e. it is not controlled by the brain. When the bladder expands to a certain level the muscles of the bladder wall contract and the sphincter muscles at the neck of the bladder and in the urethra relax allowing urine to pass. The nerves which control these actions are in the sacral area of the spinal cord.

Control of micturition is developed when a child is about 2 years old. Centres in the brain can then overrule the responses from the spinal cord until a suitable moment is found.

Under certain circumstances these processes are disturbed and a person feels the need to pass urine but is unable to do so. The bladder is distended, but for some reason the normal process is stopped. This may be because something is blocking the lower urinary tract, for example an enlarged prostate gland. This condition is termed **urinary retention**.

Diuretics

These are a group of drugs (for example, frusemide) which increase the amount of urine produced by the kidneys. They work on the nephron, changing the normal processes to enable more fluid and more salts to be passed out of the body. Caffeine (a component of both tea and coffee) acts as a diuretic as well as being a stimulant.

3: Kidney damage

Understanding renal malfunction

Because of the complexity of the kidneys there are many possible ways in which they can go wrong. We can, however, simplify the picture, by considering the three stages of normal function – in other words, the way in which the kidneys adjust the composition of the plasma.

The three stages are:

1 Removal – the mechanical process at the top of the nephron.

2 Reabsorption – the way that the substances are taken back into the bloodstream.

3 Regulation – the way that the process of reabsorption is controlled at various stages.

We can identify what the kidney requires in order to carry out each stage successfully. This enables us to:

- understand why and how renal function can be disturbed
- appreciate the relationship between the renal system and other body systems.

The next activity invites you to identify these requirements for yourself. It is particularly important to work through it because it will assist you to develop a way of thinking which is helpful in understanding physiological processes. You can then apply this understanding to care planning.

ACTIVITY 19   ALLOW 15 MINUTES

The three Rs of renal function are shown in the first column of *Table 5* below.

1   Review the work you have done so far in this unit and, using only this information, fill in column 2 by listing the requirements for each function. Use simple, non-technical language. You should aim to think the process through in a logical way, without being too concerned, at this stage, with technical detail.
    For example, when considering the removal of water and dissolved substances from the blood at the top of the nephron, you may conclude that the main thing needed here is a force to push the fluid out into the glomerular capsule. We have filled this in at the top of column 2.

2   When you have completed column 2, look at the items in it and, for each one, decide what is required in order for it to happen. List these requirements in column 3.
    Returning to the example we have just considered, there will only be a sufficient net force to drive fluid out if:

●   Hydrostatic pressure in the capillaries is greater than osmotic pressure
●   There is no opposing force in the nephron.

We have filled in the first row. Please complete the next two rows.

1. Function	2. What is needed to perform this function	3. What is needed for this to happen
Removal	Enough force to push fluid out of capillaries in the glomerulus.	1. Hydrostatic pressure greater than osmotic pressure in glomerular capillaries. 2. Absence of opposing force in nephron.
Reabsorption		
Regulation		

Table 5 Renal function

Commentary

One version of a completed *Table 5* is shown below.

1. Function	2. What is needed to perform this function	3. What is needed for this to happen
Removal	Enough force to push fluid out of capillaries in the glomerulus.	1. Hydrostatic pressure greater than osmotic pressure in glomerular capillaries. 2. Absence of opposing force in nephron.
Reabsorption	Good contact between fluid in nephron tubule and blood in capillaries.	1. Healthy, active cells in nephron tubule. 2. Intact capillaries, with good blood supply, surrounding nephron.
Regulation	1. Hormones which act on the nephron. 2. A system to detect changes in the components of the blood.	1. Healthy hormone-producing glands. 2. Functioning osmoreceptors.

You may not have used the same words as these, or included all of the possibilities.

We hope that this activity has shown how the functions of the kidney depend on and interlock with many other functions. It should also have shown you that it is possible to reason out how a fault in one function can affect many others. It is not necessary to have a very detailed knowledge of physiology to work some of these relationships out, as long as you understand some basic principles.

Relating one or two aspects of renal function back to their underlying requirements should also enable you to work out what can go wrong with kidney function. We will go on to look at this in the next activity.

ACTIVITY 20   ALLOW 10 MINUTES

Now take any one of the items in your column 3 of *Table 5* and consider what might go wrong with it, and what the effect of that might be on renal function. (Once again, only use information that you have already gained.)

Here is an example to illustrate what we mean. Activity 19 identified the need for hydrostatic pressure in the capillaries to be greater than osmotic pressure in order to drive fluid out into the nephron. What could go wrong?

The hydrostatic pressure could fall and become less than the osmotic pressure. The BP in these capillaries could be low so that it would not be sufficient to force the glomerular filtrate out. This would mean that less fluid was filtered through the kidneys, less urine was produced and less waste products were removed. The waste products, especially urea, would therefore accumulate in the plasma. This happens, for example, to a person who has suffered severe injuries in a road accident and who has lost a lot of blood. The volume of plasma is reduced, the BP falls and therefore the rate of glomerular filtration is reduced. This is one reason why intravenous fluid is given as a matter of urgency to casualties.

You might like to work your example through in the same way.

What is needed	How could this go wrong?

Commentary

Table 6 shows all the items in column 3 worked through in this way.

What is needed	How could this go wrong?
1. Hydrostatic pressure greater than osmotic pressure in glomeruli	Forces become unbalanced, so too little fluid forced out
2. Absence of opposing force in nephron	Pressure build up in nephron, due, for example, to blockage by disease or trauma
1. Healthy active cells in nephron tubule	Cells become diseased or suffer from shortage of energy or oxygen
2. Intact capillaries with good blood supply	Capillaries become damaged or blood supply reduced
1. Healthy hormone-producing glands	Hormone-producing glands fail or affected by disease
2. Functioning osmoreceptors	Osmoreceptors and/or associated nerve supply damaged

Table 6

This table suggests that there are three basic types of malfunction, relating to:

- BP and blood supply
- the nephron – its structure and function
- the control system – hormones and nerves.

Let's go back to Michael's case study and see if we can learn which of these was the cause of his renal failure.

ACTIVITY 21   ALLOW 5 MINUTES

Please look again at Michael's case study (Resource 1). What, if anything, does it tell you about:

- the cause of his renal failure

- the main effect of his renal failure, which was identified when he was first admitted to hospital?

Commentary

The cause of Michael's renal failure is not apparent from the case study. He appears to have been quite well until his kidney function deteriorated, and then he became ill rapidly. Because of this it seems likely that he suffered from **chronic** renal failure – a condition with many causes in which kidney function deteriorates gradually over a long period, without an obvious cause, or without the cause being detected. People with this condition tend to complain of vague symptoms until the failure reaches the stage where the results of kidney malfunction suddenly become dramatic. This is contrasted with **acute** renal failure, which we will consider later.

The main effect of his renal failure was **malignant hypertension**. This means very high BP (for example, 260/150 mmHg) which, if not improved, causes changes which result in death within two years. Some of the changes caused by such high BP occur in the blood vessels at the back of the eye and are visible with an ophthalmoscope.

Thus, while increased BP can cause renal failure because of the progressive change it causes to the nephrons, it is also a result of renal failure, brought on by other causes. This is because, as we noted earlier, the kidneys have several other functions in addition to regulation of the plasma composition, one being regulation of the BP.

4: Regulating blood pressure

So far, in this unit, we have been talking about the homeostatic mechanisms which control the content of water and dissolved substances in the body fluids. We have shown that such mechanisms need something to recognise changes and something to regulate the system. The physiological terms for these things are **receptors** and **effectors**.

All the mechanisms which keep the internal environment of the body constant work in a similar way. The BP level is partly responsible for the formation of intercellular fluid and thus contributes to the internal environment. The level therefore needs to be kept constant in the tissues. This requires the operation of a homeostatic system, with structures to recognise changes in BP and others to regulate BP accordingly. Since the function of the kidney is so closely tied in to BP levels, it is not surprising to find that part of this homeostatic mechanism exists in the kidneys themselves.

Recognising changes

The receptors which monitor BP in the kidney are cells which surround each arteriole just before it divides to form a glomerulus. These cells register changes in the volume and pressure of the blood just before it is filtered. They form part of a complex structure called the **JGA** (**juxtaglomerular apparatus**).

Responding to changes

Also part of the JGA are cells which produce a substance called **renin**. This is an **enzyme** – a protein which brings about a specific chemical change in living cells.

When the BP in the kidney capillaries falls for any reason, the rate of production of renin increases. You may have come across this enzyme before. It has the ability to break certain proteins into smaller fragments. Its connection with BP is as follows.

There is among the plasma proteins an inactive substance **angiotensinogen**. Renin converts this substance to **angiotensin II**, by splitting off a part of the molecule. Angiotensin II causes blood vessels to constrict. In other words, it causes **vasoconstriction**. A substance which does this is termed a **pressor**. Angiotensin II is in fact the most powerful pressor substance known and causes any small arteries it contacts to become narrower, thus increasing the BP in them.

So renin activates the angiotensinogen, thus causing the small arteries in the kidney to constrict, raising the BP. It produces the same effect on the small arteries in many other parts of the body, including the skin surface.

ACTIVITY 22

Here is another true story of an incident in nursing care. Please read it through and then carry out the exercise that follows it.

Gerry, a man in his early twenties, was rushed into the Accident and Emergency Department of a large city hospital at 3 a.m. after an accident in which his motorbike left the road and somersaulted down a motorway embankment. He was conscious and extremely cheerful but the ambulance crew were not so happy, because they could see that his right foot was badly mangled and they suspected that his injuries were severe. He had been given pain-relieving treatment on the short journey to hospital.

His BP was quite normal when he was admitted. The house officer began his examination. The young man was dressed in a full suit of leathers. The jacket was easy to remove, but the close-fitting leggings were very difficult and had to be attacked with shears. Whilst this was happening the house officer, who had just been roused from a short spell of badly needed sleep, went to get a quick cup of coffee.

The staff nurse began to cut lengthways down the outside of the leggings. She stopped when she saw that they were saturated with blood on the inside and sent a student to find the house officer as a matter of urgency. By this time she had cut from the top of the trousers to just below the knee. Suddenly a senior nurse, who was monitoring the patient, said urgently 'His BP is in his boots. Get a drip up and get the doctor back in here right now.'

Gerry had suddenly become quite silent and grey in the face. He collapsed against the side of the trolley. The senior nurse assembled a drip stand and intravenous saline at top speed and was standing holding gloves and needle as the doctor strolled back into the room. She looked at him very directly. 'I think he needs fluids right away.' The house officer suddenly came to life, Gerry was given intravenous fluid and eventually made a full recovery.

As an exercise to reinforce your understanding of the homeostatic processes which regulate BP, write an account of what was happening in Gerry's body in physiological terms, from the moment that the staff nurse started to cut away his motorcycle leathers. Bring in as much as possible of the material you have covered so far in Sessions One and Two. You should aim to write about 100 words.

Commentary

Your account of the changes in Gerry's body might have been something like this:

When Gerry first arrived at the Department his leather leggings were constricting the blood vessels in his legs, so even though he had suffered blood loss his normal homeostatic mechanisms were enough to maintain his BP and so he was not experiencing any severe effects.

When the nurse started to remove the leggings the pressure on the blood vessels in his legs decreased and so his BP fell dramatically. The effects of blood loss were suddenly apparent.

The receptors which detect pressure and volume (including the JGA) then responded. We know of two ways in which this response occurs. Firstly a feeling of thirst and, secondly, increased renin production by the JGA. The latter causes constriction of many blood vessels, including those near the skin surface, hence the normal blood flow under his skin was reduced and his skin looked very pale.

On the basis of our work in this unit, this is as far as you will be able to go in explaining Gerry's collapse. Clearly, lots of other things are happening at the same time as Gerry experiences the symptoms of shock caused by a reduction in blood volume (**hypovolaemic shock**). For the present, we are concentrating on the renin/angiotensin system.

The effect of angiotensin is to increase the BP. It does not persist in the bloodstream. It is rapidly destroyed by another enzyme which is always present there. So the effects of angiotensin will continue only if the JGA keeps on producing renin. When the BP returns to normal, the JGA cuts down its output of renin in response. In this way, the BP is kept constant under normal circumstances.

This is an example of a **feedback loop** – a kind of control system found in many homeostatic mechanisms. The components of such a system are shown in *Figure 8a*.

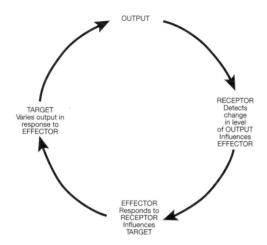

Figure 8a The components of a feedback loop

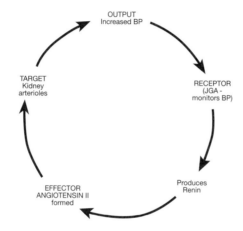

Figure 8b The feedback loop operating to maintain Gerry's blood pressure

Feedback control

Figures 8a and *8b* show the basic components of all feedback loops. They include something which detects change (the **receptor**) and something which responds to change (the **effector**) acting on something else (the **target**) to bring about a change that restores balance.

A simple domestic example illustrates this clearly. In a domestic central heating system the thermostat is the receptor. If the temperature of the circulating air changes it communicates with the boiler (the effector) through an electrical communication system. The effector then influences the targets, the radiators, which warm the air and thus cause the thermostat to switch off again.

Let's compare this with the case of the control of renal BP. In this case, receptor cells of the JGA detect changes in the pressure of the blood coming in to be filtered. They communicate with the renin-producing cells, also in the JGA, which output renin into the blood in the arterioles. This converts angiotensinogen to its active form angiotensin II. This is the effector which then reaches its target (the kidney arterioles) through the bloodstream (see *Figure 8b*).

As vasoconstriction occurs the increase in renal BP is detected in the JGA and the output of renin stops.

Angiotensinogen is present in the plasma all the time, but it is inactive until renin acts upon it. In the next activity we would like you to think about the reasons for this.

ACTIVITY 23 — ALLOW 5 MINUTES

Here are two questions which illustrate some general principles about this type of homeostatic control. Consider your answers and record them in the space below. (You may find it helpful to use metaphors to make your point.)

1 Can you suggest why angiotensinogen is present all the time in an inactive form?

2 Consider the other control systems you have encountered up to this point in the unit. Do you notice anything similar about the way in which these different systems operate?

Commentary

Your answers could have been similar to these (although we wouldn't expect you to have suggested the same metaphors):

1 Angiotensin is obviously dangerous stuff to have around, but it is sometimes needed in a hurry, as in Gerry's case. It therefore needs to be ready for action but 'sheathed' in some way – rather as one might keep a very sharp knife in the kitchen drawer enclosed in a protective case.

2 The renin-angiotensin system operates by allowing something to happen which was previously prevented from occuring. This is a method employed in several homeostatic systems. In Activity 18 you saw how ADH, which prevents water loss, can be switched off to allow more urine to be produced.

Malignant hypertension arising from faults in the kidneys is caused by increased levels of renin, due to damage to, or infection of, the nephrons. If the damage cannot be repaired, then the only way to stabilise the BP is to interfere with the process of liberating angiotensin.

ACTIVITY 24   ALLOW 2 MINUTES

Looking again at Michael's case study, can you identify the drug he was given for this purpose? Note it down below.

Commentary

Captopril is one of a group of drugs which stop the conversion of angiotensinogen to angiotensin. They are called ACE inhibitors (angiotensin converting enzyme inhibitors). If angiotensin cannot be produced, vasoconstriction will not occur and this will help to keep the BP down. You might like to draw in the site of action of captopril on *Figure 8b*, and check for yourself how this drug operates on the feedback cycle.

You have now reviewed two very important functions of the kidney and, in the process, learnt more about the important physiological principles of homeostasis and feedback control.

As if these two major tasks were not enough, the kidney also performs other functions. We will consider just one of them now, the role of the kidney in the production of the oxygen-carrying components of the blood.

5: The kidney and anaemia

The kidney manufactures several important proteins, one of which is **erythropoietin**, a hormone that controls red blood cell production in the bone marrow. When the kidneys fail this hormone is not produced, so the process of producing red cells is slowed down and anaemia results. The blood's capacity to carry oxygen is reduced: the person gets tired very easily and is not able to exert himself without becoming breathless.

6: Renal failure

Explaining the symptoms of chronic renal failure

On the basis of the work in this session you should now be able to look at Michael's case again and give a physiological explanation for most – though not all – of the symptoms described there.

ACTIVITY 25   ALLOW **10** MINUTES

Look again at the case study of Michael. List the things he experienced as his illness progressed and see which ones you can now explain in physiological terms. There will be a few items that you will not be able to explain yet in terms of the work you have done in this unit. You could if you wish prepare your answer in two columns, with symptom on one side and explanation on the other. Use a separate sheet of paper for this.

Commentary

Table 7 shows a list of those of Michael's symptoms which you should be able to understand on the basis of your work up to this point.

Symptom	Explanation
nausea	a consequence of raised urea level
tiredness	a consequence of raised urea level
vomiting	a consequence of raised urea level
breathlessness	due to increased fluid in the body
headache	from raised blood pressure or uraemia
loss of ability to taste	a result of uraemia
deteriorating eyesight	a complication of high blood pressure
marked hypertension	may be the cause or consequence of renal failure

Table 7 Symptoms which Michael experienced

The table does not include left ventricular failure, which was diagnosed when Michael was admitted to hospital. We will consider the link between renal failure and heart failure at the end of this section.

Nor does the table include lung cancer and pulmonary embolism, two things which Michael suffered but which, as far as we know, are not due to his renal problems.

One thing that is very striking about Michael's case is his survival. Not only did he outlive his original prognosis by many years, but he survived surgery and several medical crises. The case study doesn't tell us much about the nursing care which he received, but it is likely that specialised, high quality nursing made a major contribution to his survival. So, to end this session let's look at a nursing post that can play a crucial role in delivering such care.

7: The clinical nurse specialist

The post of clinical nurse specialist is relatively new. In clinical areas such as a medical or surgical ward the senior nurse is a ward sister or charge nurse and is responsible for the management and organisation of nursing care in that ward. The nursing team includes several staff nurses who take over this responsibility when the charge nurse is 'off duty'.

The ward sister or charge nurse is responsible for the nursing care while the person is in hospital. When he or she goes home nursing care is transferred to the Community Nursing Service.

The post of clinical nurse specialist has developed to try to bridge this division of care, when specialist knowledge is important to continuing care.

Renal diseases are not particularly common, and the care of patients with renal problems tends to be in specialist, regional units. This can be difficult for people like Michael, who may have to travel long distances.

A clinical nurse specialist is an acknowledged expert in one branch of nursing. She/he may have an additional qualification and will also have had several years of experience in that branch of nursing. This specialist will care for patients while they are in hospital, and while they are at home. They are also able to meet with community staff to advise them about the details of a patient's care.

Some patients with chronic renal failure enter a home dialysis programme, eventually becoming completely responsible for their own dialysis. To support this programme a specialist nurse is available either by telephone or to visit if any problems arise. She/he provides advice on diet, fluid intake, lifestyle, drugs and their side effects, and many other aspects of the treatment which the patient is receiving. This nurse also helps the person to manage the physical sites where the connections for dialysis are made in the body. She/he may also advise and teach local community staff about the nursing care the patient needs.

The main advantage of the clinical nurse specialist is that the patient has continuity of care. It means that someone the patient has come to know while they were in hospital, and in whom they have established a feeling of confidence, is still available to care for them when they are at home.

Specialist nurses work in many different areas – for example in caring for diabetic patients, those with a stoma, or those with asthma, as well as in intensive and neonatal intensive care.

The aim of any specialist nurse is to provide a well co-ordinated service to patients, and to use specialist knowledge to enhance nursing care. In several specialisms, the specialist nurse requires an in-depth knowledge of physiology in order to support the patient. This is particularly true of the renal specialist, who needs a detailed understanding of renal function, and fluid and electrolyte balance. However, this role gives rise to special problems and challenges. Resource 3 is a compilation of articles that provide background reading on the topic.

Acute renal failure

Michael's condition illustrated the way in which damaged or diseased kidneys can fail gradually over a number of years until a person suddenly finds himself seriously ill.

In other situations, renal failure occurs very suddenly as a result of interrupted blood flow to the kidney or the effects of injury, poisons, infections or mechanical blockage.

Longer if you wish to discuss it with colleagues

ACTIVITY 26   ALLOW 5 MINUTES

Here is an account of the treatment of a patient with acute renal failure. It is a true story and took place around 1980 in a large teaching hospital.

Robert had an operation on one of his kidneys in a ward specialising in urological surgery. The person who told this story couldn't remember what the operation was for. She was a student nurse at the time and this was her first clinical placement.

The ward was very task-orientated and the first-year learners had to empty all the catheters and chart the urine outputs. Since every post operative patient was catheterised, this was quite a task.

The learners were also held responsible for maintaining records of fluid intake. The senior sister was very strict, and anyone who failed to give fluids as instructed was in for serious trouble.

Robert underwent a relatively simple operation and was up and about on the second post operative day. However, his urine output suddenly decreased and he went into acute renal failure. At first he continued to take care of himself and was able to get around the ward. The nurses were instructed to make sure that he drank a tumbler of water every half hour. Robert soon became shaky on his feet, with severe headache. The nurses were instructed by the senior sister to keep pushing fluids. The second sister was heard by the student to say 'We're drowning him, but what can you do?' The student didn't understand what this meant, but did not like to ask.

Within 48 hours Robert was unconscious. He was given intravenous fluids. The student noticed that his breathing was laboured and he was coughing up pink, frothy sputum. When he died, after two more days, the second sister was very upset and the ward atmosphere was extremely tense. Robert was 52 at the time of his death.

The student thought a lot about that incident. She realised that the much younger second sister disagreed with the senior sister, who was acting on the consultant's instructions to the letter. She wondered if, by giving so much fluid, the nursing staff had actually 'drowned' Robert. And she wondered why he died in the way that he did.

What do you think about this case, both from a physiological and a nursing point of view? You might like to discuss it with a colleague and note down your responses to the following:

1 Which of Robert's symptoms can you explain on the basis of your current knowledge of physiology?

2 What nursing dilemma does this case illustrate?

Commentary

Here are some of the points you might have included:

Question 1.

- Robert's urine output suddenly decreased. Presumably this was caused by acute failure of his renal function, but the information that we have does not provide a reason for its occurrence.

- Tremor and confusion are signs of a build-up of waste products, especially urea, which would normally be removed by the kidneys.

- Headache can be produced by uraemia, and also by cerebral oedema.

- Breathing difficulties and frothy, pink sputum are signs of pulmonary oedema.

Question 2.

The main dilemma illustrated by this case is that of conflicting views about patient management. This event took place some years ago. We do not know why the consultant ordered fluid for Robert. He no doubt had his own very good reasons for doing so. The senior sister accepted these reasons. The junior sister apparently did not and the student was very confused by the whole situation.

We cannot comment on the rights and wrongs of this particular case, except to say that knowledge changes over time and that accepted practices become modified. Nurses with an understanding of the physiological principles underlying the care that they give and who keep this knowledge up to date are in a better position to contribute to the work of multidisciplinary teams.

Another important point arising from the story of Robert, is that nursing care should be reviewed regularly. If the aim of the care is not being achieved, the plan should be changed, by discussion with all staff involved.

This is the basis of the nursing process, which involves:

ASSESSING
PLANNING
IMPLEMENTING
EVALUATING

8: The kidneys and the heart

You began this unit by thinking about oedema and some of the ways in which it is caused. This led us into a study of the kidneys and some of the problems in the renal system which can cause oedema and many other signs and symptoms. Along the way you have seen how the renal system interacts with the hormonal system, the blood system and the nervous system. The idea of interaction is one we would like to emphasise. All the systems of the body work together and affect one another. So, a problem in the kidneys does not simply affect urine output; it has effects which spread through all the systems. Physiology can therefore teach us a great deal about the whole person and enable us to perform care from a holistic standpoint.

ACTIVITY 27   ALLOW **10** MINUTES

Please take a final look at Michael's case study and trace the story of his heart and BP problems. Write a short (50–100 words) summary of this aspect of his condition, and explain its relationship to his renal failure.

Commentary

Michael's story goes something like this:

- He started to feel ill in November 1979. Five months later he was admitted to hospital with malignant hypertension and left ventricular failure.
- He survived dialysis and an operation for lung cancer.
- In mid-1984 he suffered a mild heart attack.
- A year later it was necessary for him to have a triple cardiac bypass operation. He died in 1988.

Throughout Michael's story, reference is made to the difficulty of controlling his hypertension. So we see that his high BP resulted in his heart failure – to be precise, left ventricular failure. The left ventricle provides the pumping action which drives blood through the blood vessels. In patients with hypertension the small arteries are more constricted than normal, so the heart has to work harder to maintain the circulation. The amount of muscle in the heart wall increases (**muscular hypertrophy**) as a compensatory mechanism to increase the strength of the pump. (This is essentially a homeostatic mechanism – signals arising as a result of the reduced heart output trigger off growth of the heart muscle.)

If this compensatory mechanism does not overcome the hypertension, the actual ouput of the heart will be too low to drive blood right round the circulation and back into the heart. As you will see in the next session, the heart must fill properly if it is to beat in a properly coordinated way. Under the circumstances we have just described, the heart begins to fail. The enlargement of the heart makes the blood supply to the heart muscle less efficient and may result in a heart attack (**myocardial infarction**) when a section of heart muscle is deprived of blood.

We do not know how Michael's heart attack was caused. It may have resulted from damage to the blood vessels supplying his heart. These were repaired in 1985 when he had his bypass operation.

Summary of Session Two

- The volume of water and the concentration of dissolved substances in the body fluid are regulated by the kidneys.

- The kidney filters the blood by removing fluid from the plasma, regulating its composition and returning it to the circulation. The unwanted products of this process are excreted as urine.

- The removal process in the nephrons of the kidneys depends on the balance of forces in the glomerulus. If these forces are unbalanced, the filtering mechanism may fail.

- The pressure of the blood coming into the kidneys is very important for this mechanism. It is monitored and controlled by the JGA, which produces renin when the pressure drops.

- Renin brings about the release of angiotensin II, a powerful pressor substance which causes vasoconstriction and increases arterial BP. This is part of the homeostatic mechanism which regulates the BP.

- Too much renin, arising from damage to the kidney, causes progressively increasing hypertension.

- Renal failure may be chronic, progressing slowly over a long period, or acute and sudden.

- If the kidneys fail to remove water from the body, fluid accumulates and causes oedema, including pulmonary oedema which seriously affects breathing.

- Heart failure is sometimes a consequence of renal failure.

- The renal system interacts with many other parts of the body, including the heart and the lungs.

In this session you have begun to think about the close relationship between the renal system and the heart. We will now go on to develop this further and consider how problems in the circulation can also give rise to oedema.

SESSION THREE

Circulatory problems

Introduction

Perhaps the most frequently observed cause of oedema is that associated with heart failure. In Session Two you saw that one kind of heart failure – left ventricular failure – could be a consequence of renal failure. There are several other medical conditions, within or outside the heart, which also result in heart failure. Before you can explore these you need an understanding of the way in which the heart and blood vessels – the cardiovascular system – normally operate.

Session objectives

When you have completed this session you should be able to:

- describe, in outline, the structure and function of the heart

- identify the way in which blood flows through the heart to the lungs and the rest of the body

- explain the way that the heart beat is initiated and apply this understanding to supporting patients undergoing ECG investigations

- describe how the heart rate is varied to meet the changing needs of the body

- explain how variations in the heart beat contribute to the maintenance of homeostasis

- explain the relationship between the activity of the heart and the blood pressure

- identify the effects of right- and left-sided heart failure

- explain how oedema may be caused by heart failure

- outline the relationship between the cardiovascular and respiratory systems.

1: The healthy heart

This short section provides an outline of the structure and function of the heart. We have not gone into detail, but we have provided sufficient information to ensure that you understand further sections, which deal with some important aspects of **cardiovascular** physiology.

Observing your own heart

ACTIVITY 28   ALLOW **10** MINUTES

To begin this session we suggest you carry out some observations on your own heart. Sit quietly for a while and try to become conscious of your own heartbeat.

Locate your heart and describe its position and approximate size. Then locate the pulse in your wrist (the **radial pulse**) and count the number of beats per minute.

Work out how many times your heart beats in 24 hours. Note down your answer.

Finally, in your own words, describe what your heart is doing. You could relate what you observe to the work that you have done in this unit so far.

Commentary

Your observation will have related to the following facts. The heart is positioned between the lungs, slightly to the left. Its size is often compared with that of a clenched fist. It is smaller than many people imagine:

- about 12 cm long
- 9 cm wide
- 6 cm thick.

The resting rate varies from person to person. It is usually between 65 and 75 beats per minute but may be much lower in people who are trained athletes. If your resting rate is 60 beats per minute, your heart will beat 60 x 60 x 24 times every day, that is 86,400 times in 24 hours. It is responsible for the continual circulation of blood around the body. From the blood the intercellular fluid is formed (see Session One) maintaining the environment of the cells, bringing them essential food and oxygen and taking away waste products.

The driving force

The heart is the pump which drives blood through the blood vessels.

It is a hollow muscular organ with four distinct chambers. Its wall is composed of specialised muscle (**cardiac muscle**), while the inside is lined with a layer of very smooth cells which allow blood to flow with as little turbulence as possible. Surrounding the heart muscle there is a protective layer (the **pericardium**) made of tough fibrous tissue on the outside and a double layer of smooth, more delicate cells inside. Some details of the structure of the heart are shown in *Figure 9*.

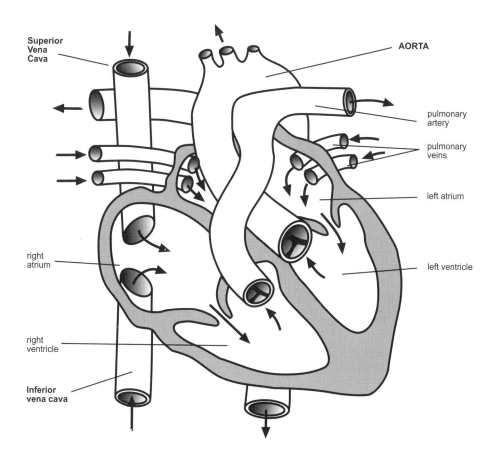

Figure 9 Section through the heart

The structure of the pericardium allows the heart to move freely inside the outer protective layer.

Sometimes inflammation occurs in the lining layers of pericardium, reducing the amount of movement that can take place and causing pain (**pericarditis**).

The continuous activity of the heart requires a very special kind of muscle. Cardiac muscle is like no other tissue in the body. It must:

- contract repeatedly throughout life and it has to contract in a co-ordinated manner if it is to act as an efficient pump

- respond to the varying circumstances in which the body is placed – at rest, during exercise, during times of critical stress, and so on.

Its structure is therefore specialised, to fulfil this very exacting role.

Pathways through the heart

Each time the heart beats it sends blood around two separate circuits. A clear picture of these is needed in order to understand the principles of cardiovascular physiology.

| ACTIVITY 29 | ALLOW 5 MINUTES |

Figure 10 is a simplified diagram which shows the direction in which blood flows through the heart. Study this diagram and then write an account of the route of a blood cell which enters the right side of the heart and completes one circuit of the body.

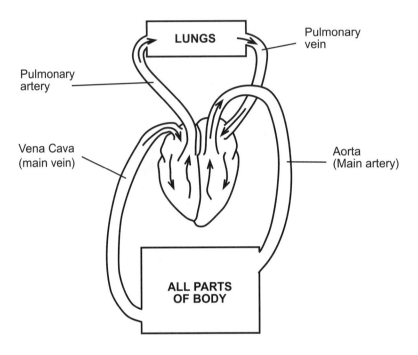

Figure 10 Simplified diagram of the direction of flow through the heart, lungs and body

Commentary

Here is the route travelled by a red blood cell from the right side of the heart:

It arrives in one of the two large blood vessels, the inferior and superior **venae cavae**. These open into the right upper chamber (**atrium**) of the heart. When this is full a valve opens and blood flows into the right lower chamber (**ventricle**).

When the right ventricle is full the muscle of the ventricle contracts and blood is expelled into the **pulmonary artery**. The blood then flows to the lungs, where the artery divides into a capillary network. These tiny vessels then join together to become veins carrying blood out of the lung, via the **pulmonary veins**.

The blood in the pulmonary veins flows into the left atrium of the heart and, again, as this chamber fills the valve between the atrium and ventricle opens allowing the left ventricle to fill. When the left ventricle is full it contracts, and blood is pushed out into the main artery, the **aorta**, from where it circulates around the body. Therefore each blood cell travels around a circuit to the lungs (**pulmonary circulation**) and a circuit to the rest of the body (the **systemic circulation**) on each complete circuit.

Although we have described the journey through the heart as if the right side and the left side are independent, in fact the two sides of the heart contract simultaneously. With every heart beat some blood is pumped to the lungs and some is pumped into the aorta to maintain the systemic circulation.

Controlling blood flow

It is clearly essential that blood flows through the heart in the correct direction. For example, when the left ventricle contracts, blood must flow out into the aorta and not back to the left atrium. This is where the valves come in. They ensure that the blood travels in the right direction through the heart. You can see how some of the valves look by referring back to *Figure 9*.

2: The heartbeat

What makes the heart beat?

The first physical examination of a person's life is usually when the midwife listens to their heartbeat during their mother's pregnancy. The heart starts beating in early pregnancy and never stops throughout the life span. What makes it start, and keeps it going? The next activity will help you to focus on these questions.

ACTIVITY 30　　　　　　　　　ALLOW 5 MINUTES

Here is a description of what happens when a person's heartbeat is investigated in hospital. It is written in the actual words of an elderly lady who was very nervous about the whole procedure. As you read it, try to imagine how it must feel to someone who is not used to all the technology. Then work out what is actually being measured during this procedure and record your answer below.

'I had these like palpitations and Dr Wilson sent me to hospital. I was under Dr Raeburn, he's a big man there. He came along and sat down on my bed. "Mrs Evans", he said, "We just want to see how your heart is doing."

'He was right nice, but he didn't say a lot. Then this young girl came along with a box and a TV thing on a trolley. I had to take nearly everything off and then she fastened these like sucker things on me with some jelly – right cold it was. I didn't know if I would feel anything. Then she plugged this trolley into the mains. I thought "Hello, I'm connected up now. Whatever's going to happen?"'

'Nothing happened though, except like a green line going up and down on this little TV, and a long piece of paper coming out from somewhere. Then they went away and had a good look at it. They left me fastened up to the machine. I didn't like to move about much, in case something came loose and I got a shock.'

Commentary

Perhaps you were able to put yourself in the position of Mrs Evans and imagine how frightening it could be to be attached to a piece of electrical equipment. Unless someone reassured her she might imagine that electric current would flow from the machine, and she might have no idea that her own heart was producing electrical activity.

This machine measures the heart's own electrical activity. The trace that it produces is the **electrocardiogram** (ECG).

Perhaps this could have been explained to Mrs Evans along the following lines:

'Each time anyone's heart beats it creates a very small electrical current. This happens all the time. The ECG machine picks up the current from your heart. We can get a picture of the way your heart is working from the shape of the green line on the machine.'

'So the machine is just picking up the usual activity of your heart. It isn't sending anything back to you, and it can't possibly give you a shock, whatever you do.'

Then the nurses might have gone on to show Mrs Evans that nothing dreadful would happen if the leads came off or if the machine was touched.

Having an ECG taken can be stressful in itself for people who already have a stressed heart. Since Mrs Evans already has a heart problem it is very important that she avoids further stress.

The electrical activity leading to the contraction of the atria measured by the ECG starts at the heart's own pacemaker (the **sinoatrial (SA) node**). *Figure 11* shows where this is located. You might like to refer to *Figure 11* as you read the following description of the generation of the heartbeat.

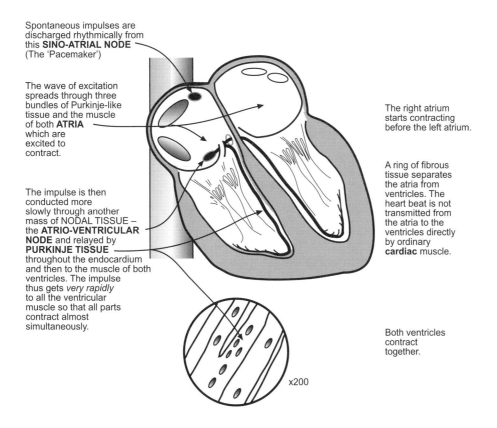

Spontaneous impulses are discharged rhythmically from this **SINO-ATRIAL NODE** (The 'Pacemaker')

The wave of excitation spreads through three bundles of Purkinje-like tissue and the muscle of both **ATRIA** which are excited to contract.

The impulse is then conducted more slowly through another mass of NODAL TISSUE – the **ATRIO-VENTRICULAR NODE** and relayed by **PURKINJE TISSUE** throughout the endocardium and then to the muscle of both ventricles. The impulse thus gets *very rapidly* to all the ventricular muscle so that all parts contract almost simultaneously.

The right atrium starts contracting before the left atrium.

A ring of fibrous tissue separates the atria from ventricles. The heart beat is not transmitted from the atria to the ventricles directly by ordinary **cardiac** muscle.

Both ventricles contract together.

x200

Figure 11 The sinoatrial node

Like all muscles, the heart muscle is stimulated to contract by electrical activity in the form of nerve impulses. The SA node generates an impulse which produces a contraction through the walls of both atria. Because of the unique structure of the heart muscle, this impulse spreads very rapidly through the walls of the atria, enabling them to contract in a co-ordinated way to push the blood down into the ventricles.

The impulse then travels down through the heart muscle and reaches another group of specialised cells (the **AV node**). When the impulse arrives it stimulates the AV node to produce a second burst of electrical activity, which travels down a track of fibres to the pointed **apex** of the ventricles. The cardiac muscle of the ventricles is stimulated to contract, starting at the apex. The contraction rapidly spreads upwards, forcing the blood out of the ventricles and into the large blood vessels, which carry blood away from the heart.

These bursts of electrical activity show up as peaks on the ECG trace. *Figure 12* shows part of the trace.

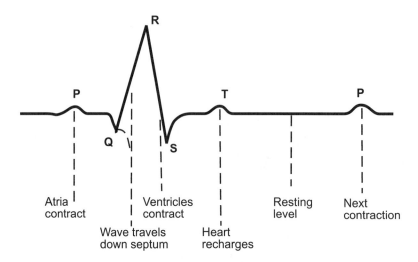

Atria contract

Wave travels down septum

Ventricles contract

Heart recharges

Resting level

Next contraction

Figure 12 The ECG trace of a single heartbeat

The peaks on the ECG trace correspond to the different stages in the generation of the heart beat.

As you noted earlier, the beginning of the sequence is stimulation of the atrial muscle by the action of the SA (sinoatrial) node. This causes the atria to contract. The '**P' wave** on the ECG is termed the **atrial complex** and represents the electrical activity leading to the contraction of the atria.

The '**QRS' wave** represents the impulse travelling from the AV node down the septum, followed by the contraction of the ventricles.

The '**T' wave** represents the process during which the heart muscle is 'recharged' before another contraction can occur. This is termed **repolarisation**.

Normally, the sequence of events begins, as we have described, at the sinoatrial node. The normal sequence is termed **sinus rhythm**. However, a rhythmic beat can be initiated from other places in the heart – the AV node or the track of fibres which conduct impulses to the apex, for example. These sites can come into operation if the connection from the node is severed for any reason – such as a heart attack. If, for example, a portion of the septum is damaged, no impulse can pass down from the AV node. A spontaneous, slower beat will arise from a point on the septum below the site of damage. This condition is called a heart block. The beat is not fast enough to keep all body processes functioning normally. A person with this condition may feel faint or collapse because insufficient blood reaches their brain.

The problem is solved by using an artificial pacemaker on a temporary or permanent basis. This is a wire which is inserted through a large vein in the right arm or right side of the neck so that it travels into the right ventricle. The wire is connected to an electronic box which produces electrical stimuli at a set rate to initiate a normal heart beat.

The cardiac cycle

The complete sequence of events occurring during a single heart beat is known as the **cardiac cycle**. If the heart is working at a rate of 75 beats per minute the cardiac cycle will take 60/75 seconds to complete (0.8 seconds).

The first part of the cycle is the contraction of the atria. This takes 0.1 seconds. As blood is forced through into the ventricles the pressure in these chambers rises and forces the valves leading to the atria shut. They close sharply, making a noise which may be heard with the stethoscope and which is described as the first heart sound.

When the ventricles start to contract, pressure quickly rises until it is sufficient to force open the valves into the arteries. Blood is forced out into the aorta and pulmonary artery. Both of these vessels, as you will recall, have elastic walls and soon the pressure in them is greater than in the ventricles, causing the valves between ventricles and arteries to snap shut. (This is called the second heart sound.) The period of ventricular contraction is termed ventricular **systole**. It lasts for 0.3 seconds.

The rest of the cycle, when the ventricles are recovering and refilling, is ventricular **diastole**.

Figure 13 shows how the pressure in the ventricles changes during one complete cycle and when the heart sounds occur.

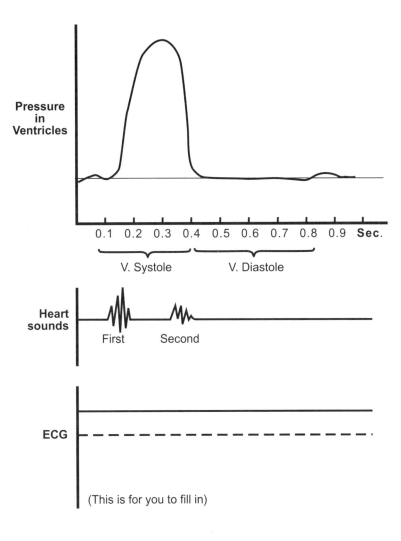

Figure 13 The cardiac cycle

ACTIVITY 31

The bottom line of *Figure 13* has been left blank. Referring back to *Figure 12*, draw in the ECG trace to fit in with the other events in the cycle.

Commentary

Figure 13a shows how the three traces correspond. The P wave occurs just before the first heart sound and the QRS wave occurs between the first and second sound, during ventricular systole.

The shape of the ECG trace which I have just described is seen when the heart is beating normally in sinus rhythm. Irregularities of the heartbeat produce an altered shape and from this shape the source of the defect or damage can be diagnosed.

One of the most serious irregularities is **ventricular fibrillation** (VF) which is seen when the ventricles are contracting in an unco-ordinated way.

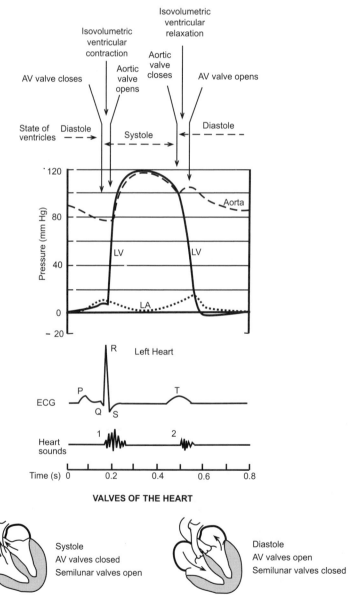

Figure 13a The relationship of the electrical activity of the heart to its contraction

Checking the heart rate

Normally, we are not aware of our heart beat. It only impinges on our consciousness when some change takes place – when the heart rate speeds up, for example. By taking the radial pulse we can observe changes in the heart rate directly.

If you attend an aerobics or other exercise class, you are probably used to taking the pulse in your neck, the carotid pulse, too. Instructors often suggest that you count your pulse for 15 seconds to make sure that you are exercising well but not too strenuously. However, this is not a very accurate way to assess your pulse rate. Multiplying an answer by four will exaggerate any error. For example, if your heart rate in 15 seconds was only 12 you would record an answer of 48 – whereas if you counted for 30 seconds you might find you had reached 27 giving a rate per minute of 54. Similarly, if the pulse is irregular a short time will not be representative of a whole minute and the calculated rate may differ from the true value.

We would now like you to investigate the way that your own heart rate changes as you go about your normal life.

ACTIVITY 32   ALLOW 30 MINUTES

You have probably been sitting still for several minutes while working on this session. However, if you have just had a break wait at least five minutes before trying this activity.

Record your radial pulse for 30 seconds after you have been sitting at rest for five minutes. (Reading A)

Now walk about the room for a minute and note your pulse again. (Reading B)

Next be energetic – for example, run on the spot for two minutes. Sit down and take your pulse again. (Reading C)

Now check your pulse every 30 seconds to discover how long it takes for the rate to return to the level of Reading A. Record your findings below.

Commentary

No doubt you observed that gentle exercise did not affect your heart rate, as measured by Reading B, very much. However, Reading C was probably much higher than either A or B, and the level gradually returned to normal. The length of the time this took depends on the level it reached while you were exercising and your own degree of fitness.

One of the aims of any exercise programme is to increase the **cardiac reserve**, that is, the ability of the heart to respond to different levels of activity without stress.

Athletes in training develop a slower pulse rate at rest and their pulse rate at peak activity is about 100 beats per minute. By comparison an unfit person would record a pulse rate of over 150 after a short burst of high activity. His or her pulse would take much longer to return to the resting level than would an athlete's.

The SA node sets the basic heart rate. The rate is influenced by external factors, such as temperature. If the core temperature of the body falls, the rate at which the heart beats also drops. However, in all but the most extreme conditions the body's homeostatic mechanisms ensure that the temperature of the heart itself remains constant.

The SA node is also subject to its own internal control mechanism, which allows the heart rate to change from moment to moment according to the level of activity of the body. Clearly this is necessary, because during activity muscles are working hard and so need increased amounts of oxygen and nutrients. This means that the heart has to beat faster to maintain the blood flow, but then must return to the resting state when activity slows down.

The heart rate cannot be controlled consciously. It changes without our knowledge and, indeed, sometimes a rapid heart rate is an unpleasant effect which we would like to be able to control.

ACTIVITY 33　　　　ALLOW 5 MINUTES

Reflecting on your own experiences, identify circumstances in which you were conscious that your heart rate was different from normal.

Make a list of them in the space below. On the basis of this list, can you suggest some ways in which your heart rate is being controlled?

Commentary

Few people report being conscious of a slowed heart rate, unless they are taking medication to stabilise the rate. But there are many circumstances in which we are conscious of an increased heart rate, for example:

- vigorous exercise
- powerful emotion
- sexual arousal.

This suggests that heart rate is linked to physical activity and to the state of the emotions. It suggests that the nervous system might be involved in the control of the heart rate.

This is, in fact, the case. The heart rate is influenced by a part of the nervous system called the **autonomic system** which controls many body activities of which we are not usually conscious.

The autonomic nervous system could be compared to the two foot pedals you use when driving a car, the accelerator which speeds you up and the brake pedal which slows you down. In the autonomic nervous system the branch that 'speeds up' most processes is called the **sympathetic nervous system** and the braking or slowing down system is the **parasympathetic nervous system**.

Nerves from both these systems travel from the brain to the heart and help to control the heart rate.

Receptors all around the body monitor the internal state and send information back to the brain so that further changes in heart rate may be made.

The two systems work together, continually adjusting the heart rate to meet the needs of the body. It was these two systems which brought about the changes which you observed when you varied your degree of exercise in Activity 32.

3: The heart and blood pressure

In an earlier session we described the important relationship between the kidneys and blood pressure. The kidneys depend on correct blood pressure for their function and they are involved in the control of blood pressure. The heart, too, is involved in the maintenance of blood pressure.

Balancing forces

A useful model for describing the way that blood flows through the cardiovascular system is that of a garden hose connected to the mains water supply. The speed at which the water flows through any part of the hose depends on the force which is driving it forward. This, in turn, depends on three things.

Firstly, *the power in the mains supply*. This is generated by a pumping station somewhere along the line.

Secondly, *factors which reduce the pressure before the water gets to the garden*. If the garden is on top of a hill, or if the main water pipes are blocked in some way, then the water pressure will be much lower than that in a house near to the pumping station.

Thirdly, *the diameter of the hose* at that particular point. If the hose is wide the pressure will be relatively low and the water will trickle through slowly. However, if the hose is narrow the pressure will be greater and water will spray out at the end.

The cardiovascular system is comparable in some ways to this model. The pressure in any part of the system depends on:

- the strength of the pump (the heart)

- the distance from the pump (or any blockage)

- the diameter of the tube (the blood vessel).

However, the cardiovascular system also has many more complex features, as we will now explain.

The heart is certainly the pumping force, especially the left ventricle, which forces blood around the systemic circulation, supplying all parts of the body except the lungs. The strength of the heartbeat determines the pressure in the vessels branching off the aorta.

It is important to bear in mind the main task of the cardiovascular system, which is to provide the intercellular fluid for all the cells of the body. Somehow, the high pressure of the arterial blood has to be adjusted before it gets to the small capillaries, and adjusted to just the right pressure to produce the intercellular fluid. This adjustment is brought about by the second feature you have considered – the distance from the pump and the presence of any impediments to the flow.

The main arteries, the aorta and its principal branches, have elastic walls which stretch and recoil as waves of blood are pumped through. The smaller arteries and the arterioles are also elastic and have muscles in their walls, so that their diameter can be controlled by contraction and relaxation of these muscles.

This demonstrates the third factor influencing pressure within blood vessels – the diameter of the vessel. A reduction in the diameter is referred to as vasoconstriction – a term you came across earlier, when studying the effects of angiotensin in Session Two. An increase in vasoconstriction puts the blood under greater pressure and makes it harder for blood to flow. The resistance to blood flow produced by vasoconstriction in the small blood vessels far away from the heart is termed the **peripheral resistance**.

So the blood pressure in the blood vessels is determined by:

1   The force of the pump (the heart) pushing blood through them.

2   The distance from the pump.

3   The size of the tubes (the diameter of the blood vessels) which creates the peripheral resistance opposing the flow of blood.

ACTIVITY 34   ALLOW 3 MINUTES

In Session Two you worked out the strength of the force driving fluid out of the capillaries into the intercellular fluid. Thinking about the way you did this, describe how you would work out the force which the blood in any vessel was exerting at a particular time. We would like you to describe this in ordinary, non-technical language.

Commentary

To find this force you would need to subtract the force opposing the blood flow (the peripheral resistance) from the force pushing the blood through (the force generated by the contraction of the ventricles).

The resulting force is what we feel as the arterial pulse. Let's think about the pulse for a while, to develop our ideas about the force which is generated.

ACTIVITY 35

You have already taken your own pulse a number of times. Now try taking the resting pulse of several other people, choosing people of varied ages, both male and female. Record the number of beats per minute for each person and describe any other differences that you can notice between them.

Take your own pulse again at rest and after exercise. Apart from the increase in pulse rate, describe any difference you notice in your own pulse before and after exercise.

On the basis of these observations, can you suggest an aspect of the heart beat, other than its rate, which varies from person to person and from time to time?

This will take as long as you need to secure five or more people who will allow you to take their radial pulses. The actual observation will take less than one minute per person, but you may need to spread the work out over several days to enable you to observe a range of different people.

Commentary

In comparing several people you may notice that some pulses are strong and full whilst others feel more feeble and 'thin'. A reasonable guess to make is that the difference is due to the volume of blood pumped out of the heart with each heartbeat.

This is indeed the case. This amount is called the **stroke volume** and its size influences the blood pressure.

ACTIVITY 36   ALLOW **10** MINUTES

Perhaps you remember that, earlier, we said that the blood pressure is the same as the hydrostatic pressure in the blood vessels. Could you now work out how the force driving the fluid out of the capillaries to form the intercellular fluid relates to the stroke volume of the heart? Review your work from Session Two and describe this relationship (in ordinary language, not numbers).

Commentary

In Activity 15 you worked out that the force driving fluid out of the capillaries was the hydrostatic pressure in the capillaries minus the osmotic pressure of the plasma.

You have just seen that the stroke volume contributes to the hydrostatic pressure, and that the peripheral resistance reduces the hydrostatic pressure in the capillaries.

So the force driving fluid out of the arterial capillaries will be due to a combination of:

- the stroke volume
- peripheral resistance
- osmotic pressure of the plasma.

What about the force driving fluid back into the capillaries at the venous end? The hydrostatic pressure here is not directly due to the pumping action of the heart but rather to the ease with which blood can flow back into the heart. If this flow is restricted by problems related to the veins or the heart, blood will accumulate in the veins, especially in lower parts of the body such as the feet and legs. The hydrostatic pressure opposes the return of fluid to the capillaries, while the plasma osmotic pressure pulls it back in. So the force driving fluid back into the capillaries is a combination of the hydrostatic pressure in the veins and the osmotic pressure of the plasma. Its strength is affected by the condition of the veins and the heart.

ACTIVITY 37 — ALLOW 5 MINUTES

You might like to read through this line of argument for a second time. When you have done so, perhaps you will agree that oedema will not occur as long as these two sets of forces are in balance. In other words, fluid will not accumulate in the tissue as long as the forces pushing it out of the arterial capillaries are matched by the forces pulling it back into the venous capillaries. In the light of this, can you work out what will happen if the hydrostatic pressure in the leg veins increases?

Commentary

If the hydrostatic pressure in the leg veins increases, the pressure preventing fluid from returning to the capillaries will exceed the osmotic pressure pulling fluid back. The net result will be that less fluid returns to the blood than is forced out in the tissues of the feet and legs. Therefore oedema results, as in Mr Granville's case.

Now that you have worked through this particular argument you should be able to work out the effects of various changes in any of the forces which govern the production of intercellular fluid. This will help you to deepen your understanding of the many causes of oedema.

To conclude our study of the healthy heart, let's take a look at the overall effects of some of the factors we have considered.

Cardiac output

You have studied, in some detail, the rate at which the heart beats and the amount of blood pumped out with each beat. These two factors together determine the amount of blood being pumped into the arteries in any given time period. This is termed the **cardiac output**.

As you have seen, the reason for the circulation of the blood is the need to maintain the internal environment of the living cells, and to supply the food and oxygen which they need. When the body is at rest, just 'ticking over', the needs of the cells are at their lowest, at least in a person who is healthy. As soon as extra work is done, even by just standing up, extra demands are made and so the cardiac output has to increase. This is why, as we exercise, our cardiac output goes up by increasing both heart rate and stroke volume.

Obviously, there is a limit to the extent to which the heart rate can increase. Ordinary people soon reach this limit. Athletes often have a natural advantage in that their resting heart rate is normally lower than average and training enables them to increase their stroke volume. So they are able to increase their cardiac output to a much greater extent than untrained people.

The heart: a physiologist's view

In this session, we have just touched upon some of the complex ways in which the cardiovascular system operates. For the next activity we provide some information which emphasises how truly remarkable this system is.

ACTIVITY 38　　　ALLOW 20 MINUTES

Please read through Resource 4. Make a note below of anything you consider to be particularly interesting. You might like to use the resource as the basis for a discussion with a group of colleagues, focusing on one of the following questions:

1 Are there similarities between the way that physiologists and nurses think about people receiving health care?

2 What is so extraordinary about the heart?

Commentary

Resource 4 provides much food for thought on these and many other topics.

1 Professor Noble sees physiological processes as being closely tied in with human history and culture. He sees the human being as more than the 'message of the genes' and therefore, according to this report, he disagrees with those biomedical scientists who view the human body as a set of separate systems.

   Nurses, from a different standpoint, view the person needing care as a whole, combining the physiological, psychological and cultural aspects of their present situation. So we could argue that these two ways of thinking show similarities.

2 There are many pieces of information in this article that emphasise the heart's 'phenomenal performance'. These include its:

   ● endurance (70 years at 60 beats per minute)
   ● superiority to any engineered pump
   ● flexibility (range of beat rate from 20 to 200 beats/minute)
   ● ability to increase output tenfold
   ● ability to work as a single muscle
   ● vast safety margins.

This summary of a leading physiologist's view of the cardiovascular system demonstrates how much is known and how much is yet to be discovered. It reinforces our opinion that we should look at physiology from a whole person point of view, rather than in terms of separate systems. We hope it will encourage you to widen your view of the subject, too.

4: The failing heart

The report you have just considered emphasises the strength and endurance of the healthy heart. However, eventually every heart will lose its efficiency and eventually cease to beat. Heart failure is evident when either the left or the right ventricle is unable to maintain the circulation which it drives.

Left ventricular failure (LVF)

If the left ventricle is unable to pump effectively the stroke volume is reduced. This has two main consequences. The passage of blood through the left side of the heart is slowed down and the cardiac output is reduced, lessening the blood pressure in the arteries.

Let's look at these in turn.

First, because the ventricle does not empty completely, blood builds up in the left atrium, causing back pressure, first in the veins returning blood from the lungs and then in the capillary system within the lungs.

There is increased hydrostatic pressure in these capillaries because the flow is being slowed, and as a result fluid is pushed out of the capillaries into the intercellular space. This is just the same process as that described in Activity 11. However, in the lungs, the intercellular fluid is very close to the air spaces of the lungs. So the fluid is forced out of the interstitial spaces and into the air sacs of the lungs themselves. *Figure 14* shows what happens.

1. IN A HEALTHY PERSON

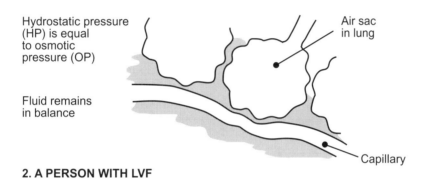

Hydrostatic pressure
(HP) is equal
to osmotic
pressure (OP)

Air sac
in lung

Fluid remains
in balance

Capillary

2. A PERSON WITH LVF

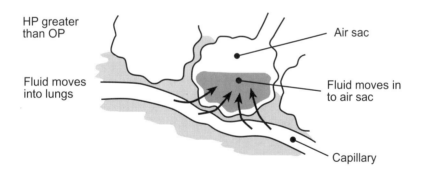

HP greater
than OP

Air sac

Fluid moves
into lungs

Fluid moves in
to air sac

Capillary

Figure 14 The effect of LVF on the lungs

ACTIVITY 39   ALLOW 5 MINUTES

Perhaps this description has reminded you of a case which you have already studied. Here are some questions to help you explore this condition.

1   Which patient described in this unit suffered similar problems ?

2   What was the reason in his case ?

3   Using your imagination, describe what it must feel like to the patient to have this fluid slowly accumulating in their lungs.

4   What is the correct term for this condition ?

Commentary

Your answers may have been similar to these:

1   Robert suffered this condition (Activity 26).

2   He suffered acute renal failure.

3   Fluid in the lungs reduces the capacity to take in oxygen and makes a person feel breathless. If only a little fluid is present, this will be rather like the breathlessness we feel on walking up a steep hill, when we are unable to take in oxygen quickly enough to supply our needs. However, if more fluid accumulates the person will feel that they are suffocating and have to gasp for air.

4   The correct term for this condition is pulmonary oedema.

In Robert's case, the oedema was caused by the failure of his kidneys to remove excess water. This increased the hydrostatic pressure in his veins, resulting in oedema in many tissues, not just the dependent ones.

The outcome of LVF is just the same in the longer term, although it does not happen so quickly as we observed in Robert's case of acute renal failure. Progressive pulmonary oedema affects a person in this way :

During the day, while he is awake and more active, most of the fluid will collect in the lower part of the lung, possibly causing very few symptoms. The situation changes at night. When he lies down the fluid moves into upper parts of the lung and starts to drain into the main air passages.

This will make the patient waken suddenly, feeling that he cannot breathe. He will be very distressed and will be desperate to reach an open window 'to get some air'.

This symptom of acute breathlessness at night is called **paroxysmal nocturnal dyspnoea**. It is a very frightening experience. Some patients refuse to go to bed in case it happens again, preferring to sleep in an armchair.

Pulmonary oedema and LVF are helped by diuretics which reduce the amount of fluid in the body.

The second main consequence of a reduced stroke volume is a lowering of the blood pressure in the arteries. This means that blood is not pumped so effectively into the organs such as the kidney. (Returning to the model of the garden hose, LVF is the equivalent of a malfunctioning pumping station.)

The reduction in the blood supply is called reduced **perfusion** of the organs. Many organs, like the kidneys, work only if they are well perfused, and reduced perfusion may damage their cells. The consequence of LVF is therefore progressive failure of the kidneys and other vital organs. So we see that failure of part of the cardiovascular system has a serious knock-on effect on the lungs, kidneys and other organs.

How the body compensates

From your knowledge of the principles of homeostasis you should be able to suggest the way in which the body might compensate for the failure of the pump which drives the circulation. You might conclude that, if the output is weak, compensation might occur by increasing the speed of the pump.

This is exactly what happens. The heart rate increases in response to the need to drive more blood around the body. A heart rate greater than 100 beats per minute is termed **tachycardia**. It is a normal response to exercise and is no problem then, as long as the ventricles are able to fill up again between each beat.

ACTIVITY 40   ALLOW 5 MINUTES

Review your work on the cardiac cycle on page 64/65 and remind yourself of how long the ventricle takes to fill when the heart is beating at a rate of 75 beats per minute. Then work out roughly how long the ventricles have to fill up if the heart rate rises to 200 beats per minute.

Commentary

Earlier we explained that, at the rate of 75 beats per minute, the cardiac cycle took 0.8 seconds to complete. Approximately half of this time (0.3 seconds) was occupied by ventricular contraction. The rest was taken up by ventricular refilling (0.5 seconds).

If the heart rate goes up to 200 beats per minutes the cardiac cycle will take 60/200 seconds. That is only 0.03 seconds. So the time available for ventricular filling is approximately 0.015 seconds – a very short time indeed.

This is the problem with severe tachycardia. The ventricles fail to fill completely and the resulting output is poor. In a healthy person whose heart beats strongly, the heart rate can increase during exercise to a certain degree without ill effect. However, a person whose heart is damaged and not pumping efficiently will be adversely affected by an increased heart rate. If the heart rate is increased over a prolonged period, for whatever reason, the left ventricle will cease to function in a co-ordinated manner. Tachycardia may progress to **ventricular fibrillation** (VF), a condition in which the muscle of the ventricle 'quivers' rather than beating strongly and regularly. This feeble, irregular movement produces very little output and so the heart must be assisted, by external cardiac massage, or given an electric shock (defibrillation) in an attempt to get its activity back to co-ordinated sinus rhythm.

We have considered the effect of failure of the left side of the heart. Now let's think briefly about what will occur if the right ventricle fails.

Right-sided heart failure

ACTIVITY 41   ALLOW 5 MINUTES

Following a similar line of reasoning to the one you used for LVF, try to work out where the problems will occur if the right ventricle begins to fail.

Commentary

Congestion will occur in the large veins bringing blood back to the heart from all parts of the body.

If the pressure in the veins is increased peripheral oedema in the ankles and the base of the spine (the sacral area) will result, and oedema will occur in other internal organs. If you have made deductions similar to these you have, in fact, described the underlying basis for the symptoms seen in right-sided heart failure. When this condition is severe, the increased pressure in the veins becomes visible, especially in the neck. The veins look very distended. Increased pressure in the abdominal veins causes fluid to be forced out of the capillaries and to accumulate in the abdominal cavity, resulting in a swollen abdomen. Fluid accumulating in this way, from a variety of causes, is termed **ascites**.

The person suffering from these symptoms is said, for fairly obvious reasons, to have **congestive cardiac failure** (CCF). This term is used to describe failure of the right side of the heart.

Coronary circulation

As in any other tissue, the heart muscle cells are surrounded by intercellular fluid which maintains their working environment. This is provided by the heart's own blood supply. It comes from vessels which encircle the heart in the shape of a crown – hence the name **coronary circulation**.

Interrupting the blood supply to any muscle renders it unable to work properly, and if the supply is not restored quickly the muscle cells die and disintegrate. This is particularly true of the cardiac muscle. If the coronary circulation is interrupted at any point the section of muscle which it supplies becomes **ischaemic** (short of blood), ceases to function and the cells die. The degree of damage to the heart depends on the extent to which the circulation is blocked.

We can now add some information to Mr Granville's case study to illustrate what happens when a coronary artery is blocked and deprives part of the muscle of blood.

Helping Mr Granville

Please read the next instalment of Mr Granville's story and consider the questions at the end.

We left Mr Granville in Activity 11, where we mentioned that his notes showed that he had suffered a heart attack in the past.

He was transferred to a rehabilitation ward after his stroke. Here he was helped to regain mobility with the goal of returning to his home in the country.

His house was a farm cottage on a steep hillside, overlooking a wide valley. He had lived there all his life, except for a period of military service. He was unmarried and shared his home with his sister, slightly younger than himself.

Although the house was rather isolated, both the Granvilles loved their home and wished to remain there together. Mr Granville was very motivated to 'get back on his feet' and go home.

He was not a very talkative person, but as the staff on the rehab ward got to know him they found that he had a fund of stories to tell and a quiet sense of humour. He never used more words than he felt to be necessary. One day he got on to the subject of his heart attack. This is how it happened, according to Mr Granville.

About three years ago, on an early spring day, he woke up feeling 'under the weather'. He had promised to help his neighbour with the lambing and was not going to let a few twinges put him off. So although his sister was a bit worried, he set off up the hill, accompanied by his dog Gwen. As he climbed the hill he felt pain in his left shoulder and his neck. 'So I sat down for a bit of a rest', he said. 'I thought it was indigestion and would soon pass off.'

But the pain did not get better, it got worse and spread up into his jaw. He felt sick and decided that he had better go home. When he tried to stand he found that he could not and collapsed against a large rock. 'I'm for it now, whatever shall I do?' he thought. Then he remembered Gwen. She had been a champion working dog in her time and was responsive to his every command. With 'a bit of difficulty' he tied his scarf round her neck and sent her home. Within ten minutes he could hear her barking outside the cottage door. His sister came out and could just make him out, slumped against the rock far up the steep hillside. 'Then it was panic stations', said Mr Granville. 'What a performance!'

The nurse who heard this story wondered exactly what had happened next. She looked back through Mr Granville's notes and spoke to the Practice Nurse at his GPs' surgery. It turned out that, due to flooding in the valley, the road up to his cottage was impassable on the day in question and he had been lifted off the hillside by helicopter and flown the 40 miles to hospital.

On arrival there, the admitting nurse had noted that he was in pain, but calm. His BP was 80/60 and his rate of breathing was 34 breaths per minute.

'I often wonder', said Mr Granville, 'just what all the fuss was about and why I felt so poorly. What happened to me to cause such pain and make it so hard to breathe?'

Suppose that you are the primary nurse, on the rehabilitation ward, discussing this episode with Mr Granville. How might you answer his questions about the symptoms he experienced on that day?

Commentary

You would need to assess just how much detail Mr Granville wanted to hear. Whatever you finally decided to say would be based on the following underlying facts about the physiological processes occurring during the heart attack. You could provide him with the answers to his questions in a non-technical way.

1 What happened? Something, probably a blood clot, blocked one of the vessels of the coronary circulation, depriving an area of the heart muscle of its blood supply.

2 Why the pain? When any muscle is deprived of blood while it is active, certain chemicals accumulate in the area and stimulate the pain-sensitive nerve endings there. We will be looking at these substances in more detail in Session Six. He suffered a **myocardial infarction**, commonly called a heart attack, resulting in damage to a section of his heart muscle. This may be fatal but, as you read in Resource 4, a person may lose a considerable proportion of the heart muscle and survive. The damaged muscle becomes hardened (**fibrosed**) and non-functional, so the efficiency of the heart's pumping action is reduced.

3 What happened to his breathing? At rest, most people normally breathe at around twelve breaths per minute. Mr Granville was starting to develop pulmonary oedema by the time he got to hospital. Since his heart was not beating normally, blood was accumulating in his pulmonary circulation, as described in Activity 29.

It sounds as if Mr Granville characteristically refused to make a drama out of this particular crisis, but that he was much more ill than he realised.

In Session Three you have seen how problems in the heart affect the lungs, which are part of the **respiratory system.** So now we have observed close relationships between three major systems: the renal, cardiovascular and respiratory systems. This illustrates that they, like all the body systems, are interdependent and so should not be viewed in isolation. In the next session we are going to look at the respiratory system more closely, as many nursing activities are concerned with the support of people with respiratory difficulties.

Before moving on to this new work, you might like to extend your knowledge of the cardiovascular system and the role of the specialist nurse by reading the article on pulmonary artery pressure monitoring, which is listed in the Further Reading section at the end of the unit.

Summary of Session Three

- The healthy heart is the driving force for the systemic and pulmonary circulations.

- Its wall contains cardiac muscle.

- The unique properties of this muscle enable the heart to beat continuously throughout life in an integrated way. The heart beat has a natural rate, initiated by the sinoatrial node.

- Impulses arising at the sinoatrial node pass through specialised nerve tracts in the heart to produce a co-ordinated process of contraction – the cardiac cycle.

- The ECG monitors the electrical activity taking place during this cycle. The heart rate is subject to nervous and hormonal control. This enables both heart rate and stroke volume to vary, thus adjusting the cardiac output to the body's needs.

- In the cardiovascular system, blood pressure is affected by many factors, including stroke volume and peripheral resistance.

- Heart failure results when either the left or right ventricle is unable to maintain the circulation.

- Left ventricular failure results in pulmonary oedema and reduced organ perfusion. This may produce progressive failure of the kidneys and other vital organs.

- Right-sided heart failure produces distortion in the veins returning blood to the heart and generalised oedema will follow. This is particularly noticeable as peripheral oedema in dependent tissues.

- The heart muscle itself is supplied by the coronary circulation.

- Reduction of the blood supply to a section of the heart muscle results in severe ischaemic pain and muscle damage (myocardial infarction).

- People who survive myocardial infarction may have damaged hearts which beat less effectively. This may progressively affects other organs such as the kidneys and lungs.

SESSION FOUR

Respiratory problems

Introduction

The lungs, the associated muscles which are used for breathing, and the structures which carry air into the lungs constitute the **respiratory system**. In this session we are going to observe the normal function of this system and gain some insight into the experience of people who have breathing problems.

Session objectives

After completing this session you should be able to:

- describe what happens during normal breathing, including the respiratory movements and the exchange of gases at the lung surface

- explain the effects of breathing difficulty, in general terms

- outline the structure and characteristics of the lungs

- describe how the rate of breathing is controlled

- understand the effects of lung damage on the pulmonary and systemic circulation

- give an account, in outline only, of the role of histamine in the normal response to damage and in anaphylaxis

- discuss the nature of asthma and its effects on people

- use your understanding of physiology to suggest how nurses can best support people with asthma and other breathing problems.

1: Breathing normally

Breathing is so natural that we take it for granted until we experience any difficulty. In the next activity we would like you to concentrate on your own breathing for a while, to gain awareness of what is happening.

Observing your own breathing

ACTIVITY 43	ALLOW 3 MINUTES

Sit quietly in front of a mirror for a while and watch yourself breathing. Think about what is happening and count the number of times you take a breath in during one minute. Then see if you can adjust your breathing rate to about 30 breaths per minute – the rate at which Mr Granville was breathing when he came into hospital after his heart attack. Note down what you observe. (Note, only do this for half a minute, and don't try it if you have any sort of respiratory problem yourself.)

Commentary

Did you observe your chest moving in and out as you breathed quietly?

It's quite difficult to count your own respiration rate because, as soon as you start to be conscious of it, it's liable to change. You may have found it relatively easy to adjust your breathing rate to approximately 30 breaths a minute, which would give you an idea of how Mr Granville was breathing shortly after his heart attack.

Perhaps as you were doing the exercise you observed that you can adjust the depth as well as the rate of breathing. So unlike the renal or cardiovascular systems the respiratory system is responsive to conscious control.

Clearly, breathing is an essential activity during which air is moved in and out of the lungs. It happens automatically but its rate and depth can be controlled voluntarily.

The reason for moving air in and out of the lungs is to bring about an exchange of gases between the blood flowing through the lungs and the air. Oxygen, which makes up about one-fifth of the air, is taken in and carbon dioxide is given out.

Exchanging gases

ACTIVITY 44   ALLOW 15 MINUTES

Or longer if you have not read this material before

If you have studied the module on biochemistry, please revise Session Five to see how oxygen is used within each living cell and how carbon dioxide is produced. If you have not studied that unit, the session is provided as Resource 5. Please read this if you need to before continuing.

Commentary

You will see that oxygen must be provided to each living cell in order for food to be completely broken down and its energy conserved in a form that the body can use. One of the end-products of this process is carbon dioxide. If breathing is affected in any way, the exchange of these gases will be affected, with serious consequences, as you will now see.

A variety of causes

There are many conditions and circumstances which affect the efficiency of the respiratory system. They include:

- environmental conditions, when oxygen is in short supply (for example, in enclosed or smoke-filled areas and at high altitudes)

- mechanical obstruction of the airways (for example, choking on a piece of food)

- obstruction caused by disease (for example, asthma and cancer in the bronchial tubes)

- many disorders of the lungs themselves (for example, pneumonia, bronchitis and pulmonary oedema).

All of these conditions affect the exchange of gases in the lungs, with results which affect all other bodily functions. To illustrate what happens we will consider a relatively common condition – asthma.

2: When breathing is difficult

ACTIVITY 45   ALLOW 5 MINUTES

Please read through the following short case study and view the situation through Susan's eyes.

Susan arrived in the Accident and Emergency Department as a 'red light job' and the staff were there to meet her.

She is a nineteen-year-old engineering student, living in a university hall of residence. She has had asthma since childhood and has become used to controlling her own medication, which she takes through inhalers.

On the evening in question she was in a club with a group of friends when she became distressed and felt unable to breathe. Her friends took her out into the fresh air, but she became increasingly breathless and frightened. She couldn't find her inhaler.

An ambulance was called and she was in hospital within twenty minutes of leaving the club.

Now imagine that you are Susan and that you have just been admitted to a medical ward via Accident and Emergency. You have an intravenous infusion in progress and you are being given treatment to help your breathlessness through a nebuliser attached to a face mask. It's now an hour since you started to feel unwell and things don't seem to have improved a lot yet. You are finding it hard to breathe in, but even harder to breathe out. As you try to force air out of your lungs there is a wheezing noise. Your heart is beating very quickly and you are just on the edge of panic. People keep coming along to look at you intently. You can hear their discussions in the background and you become even more worried when you hear someone say 'She's looking a bit hypoxic', since you understand your condition well and you are aware that this remark means that you are getting short of oxygen.

Try to put yourself physically in Susan's place for a very short time (don't do this if you have any sort of respiratory problem yourself). By this I mean try breathing in normally but breathing out very little, as if this was difficult. You could make the exercise more realistic by breathing out through a drinking straw. Notice what happens, and note this down below.

Commentary

You no doubt found that your breathing got faster and that, after a few seconds, you just had to take a big breath in and out. This was a great relief as the fresh air filled your lungs.

Susan would love to take a big breath like that, but she can't because her asthma causes the small tubes through which the air passes (the **bronchioles**) to constrict.

As she breathes in (**inspires**) the muscles in her chest wall work and the air is drawn in, but breathing out (**expiration**) is a less forceful action, so the bronchioles don't open so easily and it is difficult to force the air out. The wheezing noise is the air being squeezed through these narrowed tubes. No wonder she feels on the verge of panic.

Returning to normal

Because Susan's breathing is now so inefficient, the exchange of gases is not taking place as well as it should and the amount of oxygen entering her blood is reduced. The haemoglobin in her blood is carrying insufficient oxygen. This affects the colour of the blood and thus can be seen as a bluish coloration in places where capillaries are numerous near to the skin surface – around the mouth, for example. This **cyanosis** is caused by a shortage of oxygen in the blood (hypoxia). However, things are now starting to improve.

ACTIVITY 46   ALLOW 2 MINUTES

Imagine again that you are in Susan's condition and that you have been breathing with difficulty for over an hour. Now the medication that you are given acts on your constricted bronchioles and allows them to open up. Suddenly you find that you can breathe easily again. Imagine how this must feel.

Take a really deep breath, standing in front of the mirror. Record which parts of your body move.

Commentary

You will have noticed that your shoulders, ribs and stomach all moved. The volume of the chest cavity in which your lungs are contained was increased. The reason for this is as follows:

During inspiration muscles attached to the ribs contract – moving the ribs and breast bone upwards, while the diaphragm contracts, moving downwards. The net result of these movements is to increase the internal volume of the chest cavity.

This produces a decrease in air pressure in the lungs, so drawing more air in, until the pressure in the lungs is equal to that of the atmosphere.

During expiration the muscles and the diaphragm relax, returning the volume of the chest to normal. At the same time the elastic tissue within the lungs recoils, so pushing air out.

3: The interface between outer atmosphere and inner tissues

You should now have a clear picture of how air is normally moved in and out of the lungs. Let's move on to consider the nature of the important interface between the atmosphere outside and the cells and tissues inside the body.

The inside of the lungs is essentially 'outside' the body, in the sense that it is directly connected to the atmosphere outside. The oxygen in the inhaled air is of no use until it has crossed any barrier between the air outside and the cells inside the body. This interface needs to allow gases to pass but also to form a protective barrier against anything harmful in the air breathed in.

ACTIVITY 47

ALLOW 3 MINUTES

Have you any idea what the inside of your lungs looks like? In a few sentences, see if you can describe it. Also, think about the size and location of the lungs and the way that they expand on inspiration. Make a guess at how much air they can hold.

Commentary

You might have used several adjectives to describe your lungs – pink and spongy are two which readily come to mind. Both of these are good descriptions of the appearance and texture of the lungs, indicating that they contain many small blood vessels and lots of air spaces, and that they are elastic – they return to their normal shape after being squeezed or stretched.

The total capacity of the lungs is the amount of air they can hold when one takes a deep breath in. This varies according to a person's age, sex and lifestyle. A healthy adult man has a total capacity of about 6 litres. If he is an opera singer or a swimmer his total capacity may be greater. If he has a lung disease or pulmonary oedema it will be reduced.

The air that is taken in is drawn down through branching tubes which end in round air sacs (the **alveoli**). Blood capillaries (see *Figure 13*) are very close to the lining of the alveoli. This lining is thus the barrier which controls the exchange of gases between the air and the blood. It protects the blood, and therefore the intercellular fluid, from the atmosphere in which we live. Sometimes it is necessary to remind ourselves just how fragile this barrier is. Some people describe the millions of tiny, spherical, thin-walled alveoli as being like a froth of soap bubbles. This is not a perfect model to use, but it helps to illustrate one very important feature of the structure of the lungs, which you can explore in the next activity.

ACTIVITY 48

ALLOW 10 MINUTES

Many adults enjoy an excuse for playing with soap bubbles. Here is your chance. Make a lather with washing-up liquid in a small bowl and a similar amount of lather with a bar of soap in another. Watch the bubbles for five minutes and record what you observe.

Then take a look at the ingredients listed on the packaging in each case. What difference do you notice? Make a note of this below.

Commentary

You no doubt noticed that the bubbles produced by the soap didn't last very long, whereas those from the washing-up liquid lasted much longer. If you were able to observe closely you would see that the bubbles from the bar of soap collapsed and burst.

On the bottle of washing-up liquid you would see a label similar to this:

> Contains 15-30% non-ionic surfactants,
> anionic surfactants

There is no mention of surfactants of any kind on soap wrappers. These substances are responsible for the 'long lasting bubbles'.

In order to function properly, the lungs need the huge surface area which exists on the inside of all these tiny alveoli. Each alveolus is lined with a layer of fluid which effectively forms a 'bubble', holding the alveolus open and preventing its sides from sticking together. Like any bubble, this has the tendency to burst and collapse, especially if it is pulled out of shape.

During inspiration and expiration the alveoli are stretched as the lungs fill and recoil as the person exhales. If the alveoli collapse under these conditions it is very difficult to open them up again. The alveolar lining contains substances which act to strengthen the curved surface of the fluid and prevent it from bursting. This allows the alveoli to retain their shape during breathing. These substances, which act on fluid surfaces, are called surfactants. The naturally occurring ones, found in our lungs, are similar to those which are added to washing-up liquid to stabilise the structure of the bubbles which it produces.

Surfactants are particularly important in the lungs of babies. As soon as the newborn child takes its first breath its alveoli fill with air and must remain open if the baby is to breathe on its own. Surfactants play a vital part in stabilising the alveoli.

In the womb, surfactants are not produced until the 26th week of pregnancy. A very premature baby may be born without enough to stabilise the lungs and so, when the baby starts to breathe, the alveoli collapse and stick together. The baby so affected suffers severe breathing difficulties.

So surfactants are essential to maintain the internal surface area of the lung. However, they are not sufficient to protect the lung tissues from all the challenges presented by the external atmosphere. We'll consider how this protection is achieved shortly, but first, to put this in context, we suggest you carry out the following activity to increase your awareness of these 'atmospheric challenges'.

ACTIVITY 49

During the next few hours, as you go about your normal life, make a note of all the different atmospheres to which your lungs are exposed. Assess the number of times that the quality of the air you are breathing changes. You might like to do this as a collaborative exercise with colleagues.

Commentary

Here is a list prepared by one of the authors, describing the changes experienced during one and a half hours, first thing in the morning.

Location	Feature of atmosphere
bedroom	warm, dusty
kitchen	very warm, well ventilated
outside front door	very cold, dry
kitchen	as before
garden	as before
inside car	cold, damp later, very warm, petrol fumes
office car park	cold, foggy, industrial haze.

You may have experienced changes more marked than these, but I hope that this activity will have increased your awareness of the kinds of challenges which your lungs face day by day.

In Session One we explained how the intercellular fluid acts as a buffer between the cells and the external environment. In a similar way, a protective, buffer zone exists between the air outside and the cells at the lung surface. This zone is created partly by the upper part of the respiratory tract, the nose and the windpipe, where air is filtered and warmed as it is breathed in. So the air that reaches the lung surface has been screened, to a certain extent. Furthermore, the lungs do not empty completely on expiration. So the air breathed in is also mixed with some residual air. This process reduces the effects of changes in the conditions of the external atmosphere on the lung surface and allows the exchange of gases at the interface to proceed as efficiently as possible. As long as this happens, the levels of oxygen and carbon dioxide in the blood can be maintained at the correct levels.

However, if anything interferes with this exchange of gases, the blood gas levels may be affected, with serious consequences.

Let's return to Susan for a while to see what can happen.

The effects of breathing difficulties

Before Susan's treatment began to ease her breathing she was suffering from breathing difficulty (**dyspnoea**). This can arise from many causes, including blockage of the airways. A simple first aid manoeuvre which nurses can employ is a life-saver when the airways are blocked by some object which has 'gone down the wrong way' and caused choking.

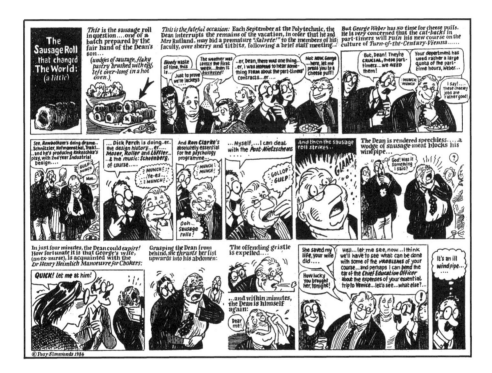

Whatever the cause, dyspnoea affects the exchange of gases at the lung surface.

As it gets worse, the effects of insufficient oxygen begin to be felt. The brain is affected and the person becomes excitable and sometimes aggressive. It is not unusual for people admitted with respiratory distress to be very irritable and even abusive to those caring for them.

The heart and breathing rate both increase as the normal homeostatic mechanisms operate to drive more blood to the tissues. Susan showed all of these effects during the period before her breathing eased. Her anxiety added to her problems as her heart rate increased under the influence of her autonomic nervous system. If you check back in Session Three you will see that we described there the problems caused by a very rapid heart rate. The ventricles fail to fill during the shortened period of ventricular diastole and therefore the cardiac output goes down, reducing perfusion of all the major organs. This can lead to fatal consequences.

Controlling the rate of breathing

When you tried to put yourself in Susan's place you might have deduced that the increase in your rate of breathing was due to shortage of oxygen. This is not the whole story, as the next activity will show.

ACTIVITY 50 ALLOW 5 MINUTES

Let's look at another person who came into accident and emergency at the same time as Susan.

Maria was admitted into the next cubicle to Susan. She had been out for the evening and her friends brought her in because, they said, she was in a state of panic. She was breathing very rapidly and deeply and was in obvious distress, complaining of dizziness and pins and needles in her fingers.

Unlike Susan, she was not given oxygen. Instead, she was asked to breathe in and out into a paper bag. This soon made her feel better and her distress subsided.

- Note down the differences that you observe between the breathing patterns of Susan and Maria when they were first admitted

- Then try to put yourself in Maria's place for a while. Breathe at your normal resting rate for 30 seconds

- Next take five very deep and rapid breaths. (No more than five, please, and once again, do not do this if you have any respiratory problems.)

- After these deep breaths let your own breathing rhythm return and observe your breathing for the next 30 seconds.

Commentary

You probably noted that Maria was breathing rapidly and deeply, unlike Susan who was taking shallow breaths and having difficulty in breathing out.

After changing your own breathing pattern to one like Maria's, did you notice that, when you stopped over-breathing, your breathing was slow and shallow for a while? Taking these very deep breaths seemed to change your automatic pattern, which then gradually reverted to normal.

So it appears that getting rid of a lot of carbon dioxide altered your breathing rate. Your body responded to the level of carbon dioxide in your blood. In fact, under normal circumstances this is the main factor controlling the rate of respiration. A moderate reduction in the level of available oxygen doesn't affect respiration. It is only when lack of oxygen becomes severe that it acts as the trigger for breathing. However, if a person has had severe lung problems for a long time, the body's homeostatic mechanisms compensate. The level of oxygen becomes the main controlling factor, so that inspiration is triggered by low oxygen, rather than high CO_2. This has to be taken into consideration when oxygen therapy is given, because if a person's respiratory system normally responds to a low level of oxygen, a raised intake will actually slow down the rate at which they breathe.

When Maria was asked to breathe in and out of a paper bag she was rebreathing her own expired air which would contain more CO_2 than the air outside and would bring the levels of oxygen and CO_2 in her blood back into balance, reducing her unpleasant symptoms and allowing her to resume her normal breathing pattern.

In studying these two young women, with their contrasting respiratory problems, you have learnt something about the effects of breathlessness, the way that breathing is controlled and the homeostatic mechanisms that maintain the balance between gases in the blood. Let's review these topics and consider some of the effects of damage to the lungs.

As you have seen, the lungs are normally spongy, flexible structures with a very good blood supply. Arterioles from the pulmonary artery divide to form a fine capillary network between the alveoli.

ACTIVITY 51

ALLOW 3 MINUTES

Thinking about the structure of the lungs, the circulation of the blood and what you have learnt about the formation of intercellular fluid, can you work out what would happen if the interior of the lungs lost its elasticity and became more rigid for any reason?

Record your conclusions in the space below:

Then think about what would also happen if the internal surface of the lungs was damaged during the process. Add these ideas to your account.

Commentary

Working from first principles you would probably conclude that it would become more difficult for blood to flow through the lungs. This would cause a back up on the right side of the heart and increase the pressure in the veins returning from the systemic circulation, resulting in pulmonary oedema. The effect will be the same as right-sided heart failure. This is, in fact, what occurs when people suffer from a chronic lung disease, such as bronchitis or lung cancer, which compromises the structure and function of the lungs.

You may have also concluded that damage to the lung surface will affect the exchange of gases, that the person will suffer from the effects of anoxia and may become cyanosed. Because of this, the respiration and heart rate increase, and the person will be dyspnoeic, finding exertion very difficult.

The lack of oxygen may affect the brain and cause the person to be irritable.

All these effects arise from damage to the tissues of the lungs. The description above is the classic picture of a person with damaged lungs.

In Susan's case, something rather different has happened. Her lungs are not damaged, since most of the time her breathing is perfectly normal. In her case the problem arises because of constriction of the bronchioles. We don't know, in Susan's case, what brings this about, but the next activity will give us some further insight.

4: What causes asthma?

Response to damage

The actual cause of asthma varies from person to person. It is often caused by an unusual response to normal environmental conditions. The mechanism for this is very complex but we can gain some understanding of the process by studying the body's normal response to damage.

ACTIVITY 52 ALLOW **15** MINUTES

Have you ever taken a detailed look at what happens when your skin surface is damaged? If not, try this activity to learn something about the normal response to trauma. This will be helpful in understanding your work in this session.

Take a pencil with a firm but not very sharp point. Draw it firmly across the skin of the inside of your forearm, to make a mark about an inch long. Look carefully at the mark over the next ten minutes and describe what you observe. Then, using only the information available in the unit so far, suggest an explanation for this.

Commentary

The first thing you will have noticed, after a few seconds, is an irregular red area spreading out from the mark.

Later you will have noticed a red line along the mark which, later still, will have become raised. The redness around the line will fade, but the raised area will persist for some hours.

This sequence of events is termed the **triple response**. It happens every time the skin is scratched or injured in some way.

You might not have described the response in the same sequence, but I hope that you observed the three elements:

the spreading redness	(**flare**)
the red line	(**red reaction**)
the swelling	(**weal**).

Your explanation for these things might have included the following points, which other people who have tried this exercise have suggested:

- The reaction and flare might be due to increased blood flow in that part of the skin. Presumably this is due to an increase in the size of the small blood vessels there.

- The weal could be due to an increase in intercellular fluid in this area. Maybe we could call this a type of localised oedema. We don't know how the fluid got there. Did it escape from the blood vessels because they were damaged by the pressure?

Histamine and the protective response

The normal response

The effects you have just observed are due to the activity of a substance which occurs throughout the body, but is particularly plentiful in places exposed to the assaults of the environment – the skin and the lungs, for example. This substance, **histamine**, causes the normal triple response which brings blood and fluid containing defensive proteins to the site of an injury, causing vasodilatation and local swelling. You are no doubt familiar with the way this occurs when one is bitten by an insect, or stung by a nettle, for example. Nerve endings in the skin respond to the presence of histamine producing the sensation of itching or pain (if large amounts are present).

Histamine has effects on a wide range of tissues. (You have previously encountered other substances with this characteristic, including angiotensin which causes vasoconstriction whenever it encounters small blood vessels, and adrenaline, which has a variety of effects.) In the general circulation histamine produces vasodilatation. This may result in headache as the blood vessels in the brain surface expand. In muscles which are not consciously controlled (as in the bronchioles and the digestive system) it increases the tendency to contract, so a person who is given a large dose of histamine will show all the above effects, including breathlessness as the bronchioles constrict. Under normal circumstances its function is protective, and it is released in the body in small amounts. However, in some people it may be produced in larger quantities when it is not needed.

Abnormal sensitivity

There are people who are abnormally sensitive to substances which are usually quite harmless (they are **allergic** to these substances). In an allergic reaction, the combination of these substances with proteins on the surface of some cells causes the localised release of histamine. This sort of reaction may sometimes be very troublesome – for example, in the case of hay fever, where the effects of histamine release are, in a sense, out of control. The next activity describes a more extreme example of the same experience.

Read the following short case study, and, as each symptom is described, think about the effects of histamine and give a brief explanation for what occurred.

George attended hospital as an out-patient for an X-ray investigation. This involved the injection of a dye into his bloodstream, through an intravenous infusion (IVI). The progress of the dye round his body would be followed by a series of X-ray pictures, providing information to help with diagnosis of his condition.

When he was settled on a bed in the X-ray department the IVI was set up and the dye injected. Five minutes later, the nurse monitoring his condition noticed that his face was flushed. George complained that he was too warm, then that his skin was itchy. He tried to loosen the neck of the gown he was wearing, saying that it was choking him and he couldn't breathe. By this time he felt seriously uncomfortable.

The doctor who had administered the dye was nearby and came to George's bedside quickly when called. He gave an antihistamine drug and some adrenaline, directly into George's circulation through the IVI. He explained that George had suffered an allergic reaction to the dye – something that occurs in a very few people.

Commentary

Here are the things that George experienced. They are all different effects of the release of unusual amounts of histamine, produced during an allergic reaction.

Symptoms	Effect of histamine
Sensation of warmth and flushed skin	Vasodilation
Itching	Stimulation of nerve endings
Constriction of the throat	Oedema in the facial tissues
Breathlessness	Bronchoconstriction

Notice how quickly these things happened. If a person who is allergic to a particular substance is exposed to it, the response happens very quickly, as histamine is released throughout the body.

Notice too, that George was given two drugs: antihistamine which, as its name suggests, counteracts the effects of histamine, and adrenaline. The latter is given because one of its many effects is to relax the muscles of the bronchioles (bronchodilatation) and so to rapidly relieve dyspnoea.

When people are in situations where there is a possibility of an allergic response, adrenaline should always be available for this rare emergency – for example, when people are receiving injections such as antitetanus shots.

Allergy and asthma

Some people who suffer from asthma are clearly allergic to things in the environment – such as smoke, house dust, cats and so on. Wherever they encounter these things, histamine-like substances are released in their lung tissues and cause bronchoconstriction, producing breathing difficulties.

Other people with asthma do not show such a clear pattern of response. Many things bring on an attack – emotion and cold conditions for example. So the situation is more complex than an allergic response and the widely available antihistamine drugs are not effective in all types of asthma. However, the principle is the same – some factor in the environment causes an abnormal response in the lungs, releasing substances which cause the bronchioles to go into spasm.

Coping with asthma

Treatment of an attack is directed towards causing the bronchioles to dilate, providing sufficient oxygen and minimising effects on the heart until the attack subsides. However, the main focus of management is prevention and support, as you will see in the next activity.

ACTIVITY 54   ALLOW **10** MINUTES

The complexity of asthma management is highlighted in the study of patients' experiences, which is provided as Resource 6. This is a good account of the impact of this illness on everyday lives and outlines how nurses can support families affected by the condition.

Please read through this resource and select as your subject one of the three people described.

Then imagine that you are a nurse working in the community, and you have visited this person to talk to them about their situation. They ask you 'Why should I bother with these inhalers when I am not having an attack?'

Work out how you would respond to this particular question.

Commentary

John is too young to ask the question, but his mother might have asked it for him, especially as he has suffered some side effects. It seems that his attacks can be severe and he becomes cyanosed. You could explain what this means and emphasise the importance of preventing the attacks.

Peter is a bit older and his symptoms seem better controlled. Maybe he can begin to understand that, as long as he prevents the acute attacks, he can do more of the things that he wants to do.

Mary is very worried by her situation. It sounds as if she has cause for concern and her risk of a life-threatening attack is considerable. Several of the strategies listed on the last page of Resource 6 could help here – discussing the reasons and triggers for her attacks, considering the side effects of the drugs, working out how much flexibility is appropriate, discussing the place of nebulisers in management, arranging practical help, and providing emotional support.

The title of this Resource, 'Asthma – a hidden disease of our times', is a very good description of the condition. It is hidden because its impact is not always understood and because the mechanisms by which it is caused are often obscure.

We hope that the work in this session has increased your understanding of the way the lungs work, the homeostatic mechanisms involved in controlling breathing and the important relationship between the respiratory and cardiovascular systems. In Session Three we explored the link between the renal and cardiovascular systems, so I hope that you can now appreciate how closely connected all three are and how a lack of balance in any one can have widespread effects through them all.

Summary of Session Four

- Normal breathing provides oxygen for cellular function and removes carbon dioxide from the blood.

- There are many potential causes of respiratory distress.

- The interior of the lungs is a vulnerable interface between the atmosphere and the tissues.

- Dyspnoea produces hypoxia.

- Homeostatic mechanisms operate to counteract hypoxia by driving blood more quickly around the circulation.

- The rate of breathing is normally controlled by the level of carbon dioxide in the blood. In people with chronic respiratory problems, this mechanism is replaced by control in response to the oxygen level in the blood.

- Histamine is present in areas of the body exposed to the environment. It causes defensive reactions to damage.

- Allergic individuals overreact to some environmental challenges.

- Asthmatic attacks are the result of bronchoconstriction in response to the production of histamine-like substances in the lungs.

Control and integration

Introduction

In previous sessions we have emphasised how three of the major body systems affect one another. We have also touched on the relationship with hormones and nerves. The subject of this session is the way in which all body systems are regulated so that they work together to achieve homeostasis.

Once again, this is something that is so much part of our everyday experience that we take it for granted. Maybe we need to remind ourselves of what the body's homeostatic mechanisms are doing, moment by moment.

Session objectives

After completing this session you will be able to:

- describe the role of the thyroid hormones in the control of temperature

- discuss the contribution of the nervous and hormonal systems to the maintenance of temperature homeostasis

- explain how heatstroke, pyrexia and hypothermia are brought about

- outline the regular manner in which body temperature varies during the day

- apply your knowledge of variations in body temperature to the provision of care.

1: The need for integration

The changing environment

ACTIVITY 55   ALLOW **60** MINUTES

During the next hour, whatever you plan to do, note down all the large or small environmental changes that happen as you go about your normal life.

Commentary

Whatever you did during that hour there would be hundreds of environmental changes for your body to cope with. You probably noticed only a few of them, such as moving from a warm room to a colder one (change in temperature), going to the lavatory (change in volume of body fluid), falling asleep (change in energy demand) and so on. But no two seconds in the day are exactly the same, as far as the demands on your body are concerned. Even glancing from left to right across the page as you are reading uses some energy, produces some heat and liberates some CO_2.

Maybe during the observation hour you experienced some major environmental changes. You might have gone from a cold, windy street into an overheated hospital ward, or from a very busy working environment into somewhere calm and quiet. Although you will be conscious of the stresses imposed by these larger changes, your body adjusts to them in just the same way as it does to the less noticeable ones.

Coping with change

The body of a healthy person needs to make all these adjustments. Normally it can absorb all the challenges which it encounters. When something out of the ordinary occurs the body's homeostatic mechanisms operate to protect its most vital parts – particularly the brain and the heart, possibly at the expense of other systems. The symptoms of hypovolaemic shock, which were discussed in Activity 22, result from the way that the circulatory system is adjusted to secure adequate perfusion of the heart, brain and other vital organs by diverting blood from the peripheral circulation.

In our discussion of oedema we have considered a number of ways in which the distribution of body fluid is controlled. These include hormones, such as ADH, and parts of the nervous system, such as the osmoreceptors. These control mechanisms result in several body systems working together in an integrated way to achieve fluid balance. So we have a dual control system achieving integration of a physiological process. This is true of all aspects of homeostasis.

In order to clarify the way that the nervous and hormonal systems exercise control I want you to consider a situation in which the control pathways are rather less complex than those for the control of body fluid volumes. Let's look at a system which involves hormones produced by the thyroid gland.

2: The function of the thyroid hormones

ACTIVITY 56   ALLOW **10** MINUTES

As an aid to understanding the functions of the thyroid hormones, we would like you to study two contrasting case studies.

The first returns to Mr Granville. We last encountered him in the rehabilitation ward. Now please read the rest of his story.

Mr Granville spent two weeks on the rehabilitation ward. During that time his condition improved, his fluid balance was stabilised and, as a result of good multidisciplinary care, he became sufficiently mobile to go back to his hillside cottage.

He lived there for five years, visited by members of the primary health care team. For the first two years he was out and about on the hills, more slowly than before but still able to take a lively interest in the neighbouring farms and local affairs. Then he began to 'slow up a bit', as his sister said.

About this time, Miss Granville became unwell. Like her brother she was a very hardy person and made light of 'aches and pains'. She began to have severe headaches and, when she finally saw her GP, she was found to have an inoperable tumour. She died three weeks later.

This was a great shock to Mr Granville. He became even quieter than before, but insisted that he would stay where he was. Community nurses, visiting regularly, noticed that he was not regaining his former interests. At first it was thought that he was going through a very prolonged period of grief.

Two years after his sister died his mental state began to get worse and he ceased to go out altogether, complaining that he felt the cold. This had never concerned him before. He even neglected to feed the dog. The GP wondered if his thyroid function was failing and arranged for him to go into hospital for tests.

Mr Granville didn't want to go, even though the ambulance was arranged. When the ambulance driver arrived at 8 a.m. it took her half an hour to persuade him to get into the vehicle.

On that day the weather was cold and windy. Mr Granville said he was 'chilled' when he eventually got into the ambulance and, although the heater was on, he complained of cold throughout the journey. When they arrived at the hospital the nurse who admitted Mr Granville found that his temperature was well below normal at 35.5 °C. The tests were abandoned for that day and steps were taken to monitor his temperature as he was nursed in a warm side ward.

When Mr Granville was well enough he was taken for thyroid function tests and the GP's suspicions were confirmed. His symptoms were the result of reduced output of thyroid hormones.

Now please read this short account of a person with a contrasting problem – an overproduction of thyroid hormones. As you read it, compare this person to Mr Granville and see if you can deduce what the thyroid hormones regulate. Make brief notes of your conclusions in the box below.

Mrs Patel has always been one of those lucky people with lots of energy. She had travelled widely as a young woman and now, at the age of 38, she manages a full-time job and a family of three teenage children with ease.

However, recently she has been finding herself more than usually irritable and tense. Sometimes her heart seems to race and she has difficulty getting to sleep. She has never been overweight, but now she is thinner than she would like to be. The most troublesome thing for her is that she can't bear to be in the kitchen – the warm atmosphere seems intolerable and makes her sweat profusely. She is worried that she is in for an early menopause.

Commentary

You might have identified that Mr Granville and Mrs Patel differed in their:

- mental alertness
- energy level
- body temperature.

So you might deduce that the thyroid hormones are concerned with the production of energy for work and heat in the body, and also that they influence the brain in some way.

Perhaps, before looking at the way these hormones operate, you might like to consider the way that your own body temperature varies throughout the day.

Diurnal rhythms

ACTIVITY 57

Take your own temperature at two-hourly intervals throughout the day and plot it on the chart below.

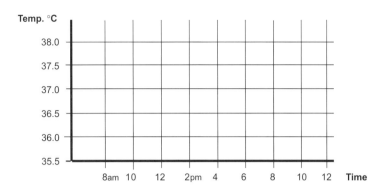

You will need to carry out this activity at intervals in the course of a day (You may if you wish continue now with the text following the commentary and return to consider the results of this activity once your record is complete.)

Commentary

Most people find that their temperature varies in a regular way throughout the day and night. If you had taken your temperature right through 24 hours you would have observed a pattern like the one shown in *Figure 15* with a low point at around 0400 hours. This is the time when many people working night shifts feel most tired. After the early hours, the temperature rises and fatigue often lessens.

Clearly, this can be a difficult time for patients, too, and we need to be aware of the particular stresses of this low point for people who are unable to sleep, in hospital or at home.

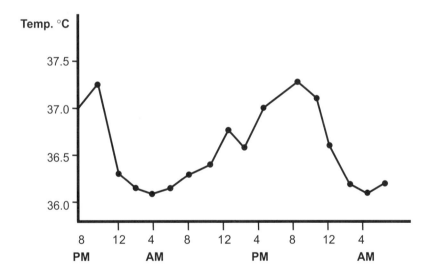

Figure 15 Temperature variation throughout 24 hours

This fluctuating pattern is termed diurnal variation. Similar patterns are found for many other aspects of our physiology, both on a daily basis and in longer cycles. People doing shift work have to cope with readjustments to their diurnal rhythms.

Thyroid hormones

Let's return to the function of the two thyroid hormones. These exert their effect on body temperature by controlling the speed at which the metabolic processes in the body work – the **basal metabolic rate (BMR)**. People over-producing them, like Mrs Patel, have a high BMR, burning up their food to produce lots of energy and body heat.

On the other hand, those like Mr Granville are not generating enough heat to keep themselves warm because they have a low level of circulating thyroid hormones.

Thyroid hormones are produced in the thyroid gland, which is the largest **endocrine** gland (weighing about 20g) and situated in the neck. Endocrine glands produce hormones which pass directly into the bloodstream. All the hormone-producing tissues in the body constitute the **endocrine system**.

The two thyroid hormones (THs) are termed T3 and T4. They both contain iodine. They are stored in the gland until required. Their release is brought about by another hormone, **thyroid stimulating hormone (TSH)**, from another endocrine gland, the **pituitary** gland at the base of the brain. They have very wide ranging effects on many parts of the body, including, for example, the nervous system. In our case studies this is demonstrated by the differences in the mental states of Mr Granville and Mrs Patel. However, in this session we are studying the thyroid hormones as an example of the way in which hormones and nerves work together, so we will just think about one of their many activities, their role in temperature regulation.

Thyroid hormones act on most body tissues to increase the rate of chemical activity – the metabolic rate – and therefore to increase temperature.

The control of body temperature

When it is cold a chain of events starts which leads to the release of thyroid hormones and the manufacture of new stores. The chain begins in a region of the brain termed the **hypothalamus**, at the base of the brain. In this area, there are receptor nerve cells which are sensitive to the temperature of the blood which flows through the brain. Some of them are sensitive to an increase in this temperature and some are sensitive to a decrease.

If a person is cold, and the temperature of the blood drops, even slightly, the receptor nerve cells which detect temperature reduction initiate the production and release of a hormone (**thyrotrophin releasing hormone, TRH**) in the hypothalamus. This hormone is therefore produced in the actual nervous system.

The pituitary gland is very close to the hypothalamus. The two structures are connected through very short vessels which convey blood directly from the hypothalamus to the pituitary. TRH travels along the short route and influences the activity of the pituitary. So at this point we have a very close physical relationship between the nervous and endocrine systems.

The effect of TRH on the pituitary is to increase the output of TSH. However, if the blood contains high levels of circulating thyroid hormones, the output of TSH will not increase, demonstrating again the principle of feedback control.

ACTIVITY 58   ALLOW 10 MINUTES

Figure 16 is a diagram of the relationships which we have just described. The solid lines summarise what happens when the body is challenged by cold conditions. Start at the point numbered 1 in *Figure 16* and trace the sequence through to remind yourself of what happens.

The dotted lines summarise what happens as the body warms up. The first of these is labelled 8 on the diagram. Trace this sequence round and label the dotted lines at points 8 through to 14.

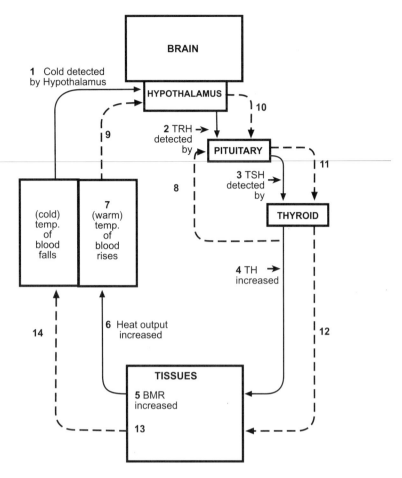

Figure 16 The hormonal control of body temperature

Commentary

Here is one way in which you could have labelled the diagram:

    8: Increased TH detected by pituitary

    9: Increased temperature of blood detected in hypothalamus

    10: Output of TRH reduced. Detected by pituitary

    11: Output of TSH reduced. Detected by thyroid

    12: Output of TH reduced

    13: Reduction in TH causes fall in BMR

    14: Fall in BMR causes reduced heat production

This diagram should have demonstrated two things. Firstly, how the body's temperature can be adjusted by the control of BMR, through release of thyroid hormone. Secondly, the close relationship between the brain and this part of the endocrine system. When you charted your own temperature in Activity 57 you observed that it followed a diurnal cycle. This is because there is a diurnal cycle in the brain, which affects the output of TRH. Human beings are normally active during daylight and asleep at night. The way that our brains work reflects this pattern of activity and we hope that you can now begin to see how this happens – when the brain is at rest there is also a reduction of heat production in the body.

The pituitary gland is sometimes called the 'master gland' because it produces a number of hormones which influence many other endocrine glands.

It is involved in long-term developmental functions, such as growth and reproduction, and the body's natural cycles. It is evident that environmental factors such as stress, sleep patterns and day length affect these functions partly through the link between the nervous and endocrine systems. The connections are not yet very well understood in humans, but what we do know about them should perhaps encourage carers to pay more attention to the maintenance of patients' natural rhythms during the process of care.

Dual control

In addition to the automatic control of temperature through the BMR exerted by the hormonal system, which we have just described, healthy people have other ways of responding to cold. If you are suddenly exposed to a drop in temperature you will take conscious action to reduce the effects and several automatic responses (such as shivering, which generates extra heat) will occur. So the nervous system, too, is involved in temperature control.

We could say that the hormonal system is responsible for the underlying, long-term control of the BMR and the nervous system deals with the moment-by-moment changes. This is something of an oversimplification, but it illustrates the general principle of the ways in which hormonal and nervous control systems operate.

You have considered the way in which the temperature control systems operate, let's now go on to think about what happens when they malfunction.

3: Pyrexia and hypothermia

You will probably notice, among your friends, that some people 'feel the cold' and some do not. If you repeated the exercise in Activity 57 with a large group of healthy people, you would find that the variation in temperature for each person was different and centred on a different baseline. Each person has their own thermostat in the hypothalamus (just as we all have our own pacemaker) and its setting varies from person to person and throughout life.

Resetting the thermostat

During certain illnesses the thermostat setting is disturbed. When it is set too high, the person experiences **pyrexia** – that is, a raised temperature.

ACTIVITY 59	ALLOW 10 MINUTES

Most people will, at some time in their life, have experienced an episode of pyrexia. Reflecting on your own experience, write a brief account of such an episode and try to give an explanation, in physiological terms, of what you experienced. Use a separate sheet of paper for this.

Commentary

Here is an account given by someone who developed a chest infection. Perhaps your description contains some similar features.

'I had a minor cold which seemed to be getting better. Then I started to feel very shivery and my legs were wobbly. I really needed to go to bed. I took some aspirin and had plenty to drink, which made me feel rather better. I could not face food.

My temperature went up to 38.5 and for two days I felt quite ill. My mother was very good – she kept coming along with a face cloth to sponge me over, and lots of drinks. Then I started sweating – I had to keep changing my pyjamas and the bed clothes. Then I began to feel like eating again.'

What was happening here? This person's thermostat was reset by the infection. It was set to a higher than normal level, so that his body acted as if he was cooler than he should be. So he experienced the sensation of cold and shivered. Because of the extra heat production his body temperature increased. His normal mechanisms for losing heat were not working.

After two days he overcame the infection and his thermostat was reset to normal. So his body now registered that he was 'too hot' and the normal homeostatic mechanisms came into play: he started to sweat. This brought his temperature down to nearer normal and he began to feel better.

In the case we have just described the 'resetting' of the thermostat was due to the presence of the bacteria causing the chest infection. Many infectious organisms contain substances which affect the receptors in the hypothalamus, directly or indirectly. Similar substances are produced by malignant tumours and from tissue destruction (such as occurs after a heart attack). In all these cases, the heat-sensitive cells in the hypothalamus are affected, causing an increase in the production of heat (for example, by increasing BMR) and a decrease in heat loss. The result is pyrexia.

Aspirin and other **antipyretic** drugs block this effect and can therefore be used to bring the temperature down to its normal level, somewhere between 35.9 and 37.4 degrees C.

Nurses are very much involved in the monitoring of temperature and the care of people who are pyrexial. Perhaps less attention is given to the problem of low temperature, but, as the next activity shows, this is an important issue in many clinical areas.

Inadvertent hypothermia

ACTIVITY 60 ALLOW 30 MINUTES

Please read Resource 7. This relates some of the theoretical work you have been doing to the clinical situation in theatre and recovery. After reading the journal article, try the following exercises:

1 Compare the maintenance of body temperature with the maintenance of intercellular fluid volume which was described in Sessions One and Two. In what general way are these two processes similar?

2 Make a list of factors which could contribute to the occurrence of hypothermia in a patient undergoing surgery.

3 Which of these factors might contribute to the occurrence of hypothermia in an elderly person, living alone at home or being cared for in a hospital ward?

4 Next time you care for, or observe the care of, an elderly person, review the extent to which these factors have been taken into consideration.

Commentary

1 The main similarity between these two homeostatic systems is that they both involve a balance between inputs and outputs. In the case of body temperature, the balance between heat input and heat output is critical.

2 The article contains a comprehensive review of the factors. These include:

- reduced food intake before surgery
- inactivity as a result of anaesthesia
- vasodilatation caused by anaesthetic drugs
- use of cold skin preparation agents
- ambient room temperature
- body type
- depression of the nervous thermoregulatory centre
- exposure of the body
- lack of sufficient insulation for the body
- administration of cold intravenous fluids
- patients' age and ability to produce heat.

3 Apart from the factors directly related to surgery and anaesthesia, most of the above are potential causes of hypothermia in elderly people.

The list does not contain a direct reference to thyroid function. However, reduced output of thyroid hormones can occur gradually over a period of years, and may remain undetected in elderly people. If a person suffering from this condition (**hypothyroidism**) is subject to some of these other factors, he or she may become hypothermic very rapidly.

4 We cannot predict what situation you will observe, but we hope you will find it interesting to check the extent to which these factors, and the risk or possibility of hypothermia, are taken into account when assessing the care needs of an elderly person.

Overcoats and refrigerators

Human beings are thought to have originated in warm climates, where their lack of body hair and upright stance enabled them to cool easily. So, in a sense, the human body is at home in a warm environment.

Under warm conditions, mechanisms to protect against over-heating are essential. If the temperature of the internal organs rises the rate of metabolism increases, because all metabolic processes work faster at higher temperatures. This accelerates heat production in the body and so a vicious circle is set in place which may end in fatal heatstroke unless external cooling is applied. So it is not surprising to find that we have well-developed automatic systems for dealing with overheating.

Clearly, people are much less at home in cold climates. To survive there we have to do more than rely on the automatic systems. It is only by making use of clothing and shelter that human beings can live in cold climates.

So we can adapt to cold by changing behaviour, whereas we need to rely much more on inbuilt responses to cope with heat. Hence the saying that 'An overcoat is easier to design and wear than a refrigerator'.

Measuring temperature

In order to review the work of this session, let's conclude by considering some of the practicalities of measuring a person's temperature.

ACTIVITY 61 ALLOW 15 MINUTES

Please answer the following questions:

1 Where is the body's temperature-regulating centre located?

2 Is the blood reaching this centre likely to be at the same temperature as the blood flowing through the vessels on the lining of the mouth? Please explain the answer that you give.

3 How long does a clinical thermometer take to reach a constant temperature in the mouth?

4 Suppose you found Mr Granville in a collapsed state at home. What might you do to help him while waiting for assistance to arrive?

Commentary

Your answers to these questions should be similar to these:

1 The temperature-regulating centre is in the hypothalamus, at the base of the brain.

2 Blood reaches this centre from the left side of the heart and its temperature reflects the core body temperature. The inside of the mouth is more affected by the environment so it may be cooler than the core, if the mouth has been open, or it could be warmer if the person has recently had a hot drink.

3 If you didn't know the answer here you might like to verify that it takes 3–4 minutes for the clinical thermometer to reach a constant temperature.

4   Knowing Mr Granville's history of poor thyroid function you might suspect hypothermia. You could take his temperature with care. (The axillary temperature might be more appropriate than the oral temperature.) If his temperature was below 35 degrees centigrade you could take steps to insulate and warm him (a space blanket or survival bag would be ideal).

The control of temperature has illustrated the way that the nervous and endocrine systems work together to achieve long- and short-term control of this component of the internal environment. In the same way, all the other features of this environment are subject to this type of control. In general, the short-term, moment-by-moment changes are mediated by the nervous system while the slower, longer-term changes, including those associated with growth, development and reproduction, are under the control of the endocrine system.

In the last session of this unit we will focus on the interface between the nervous and endocrine systems and on its relationship to the phenomenon of pain.

Summary of Session Five

- The human body can adjust to a wide range of environmental challenges. This is brought about by the combined action of the nervous and hormonal systems, integrating all physiological processes.

- The thyroid gland produces hormones with effects on many parts of the body. One effect is on the basal metabolic rate (BMR).

- Increased thyroid hormone causes accelerated BMR and increased body temperature.

- The action of the thyroid gland is closely linked to the heat-regulating centre in the brain (the hypothalamus) through the pituitary gland.

- The level of circulating thyroid hormone is subject to feedback control.

- Body temperature is controlled by both nervous and endocrine mechanisms.

- In pyrexia the hypothalamus thermostat is affected.

- In hypothermia the core temperature falls and this may affect the vital organs.

- Good technique is important in monitoring temperature.

- Nurses have an important role in the monitoring of temperature and the restoration of normal levels.

SESSION SIX

Hormones, nerves, feelings and pain

Introduction

In this session we would like you to build on your previous work to increase your understanding of the physiology which underlies many of the things experienced by people who need care.

First we will take a look at the adrenal gland, which, like the pituitary gland, is a bridge between the nervous and hormonal systems. Then we will discuss the way in which nerve impulses travel and how chemical transmission occurs. This will lead to an extended section on pain and the experience of pain.

Session objectives

After completing this session you will be able to:

- describe how adrenaline is produced and affects several body systems
- outline the relationship between adrenaline and the sympathetic nervous system
- explain how a nerve impulse travels along a nerve fibre
- outline how neurotransmitters work
- draw a simple diagram of a neuron
- recognise the signs which show that a person is afraid
- understand the causes of 'everyday' pain
- describe how referred pain is caused
- explain how painful stimuli can be modified in the nervous system
- outline the role of the nurse in caring for people suffering from acute and chronic pain
- relate the possible consequences of prolonged stress to patient care.

1: Bridging the control systems

In Session Five you observed the close relationship between the hypothalamus, the pituitary gland and the control of temperature through the thyroid hormones. This demonstrated the way that the two control systems work together.

We would now like to develop this idea further, to show how physiological processes link to our environment and our emotions. We will do this by examining the way that another gland, the adrenal gland, functions at the interface between these systems.

The adrenal medulla

The adrenal gland is located close to the kidneys. It produces hormones which are discharged directly into the blood and travel round until they reach their targets. It is therefore an endocrine gland.

The adrenal gland secretes several hormones but we are only going to consider one of them at this point – **adrenaline**, which is produced by the **adrenal medulla**.

This part of the gland is different from other endocrine tissues in that it is directly controlled by the sympathetic nervous system. This is why we have described this gland as a bridge between the nervous and endocrine systems.

The sympathetic nerve controlling the adrenal medulla arises in the brain and is responsive to many external stimuli and internal emotions. Let's look at an example of its response to an emotional state.

Fear and panic

ACTIVITY 62   ALLOW 5 MINUTES

One of the strongest emotions which we possess is fear. It is useful when it makes us flee from actual danger, but may sometimes be counterproductive if we panic. Often we experience a similar emotion when we are in no real danger, but faced with a difficult situation, such as an exam or a job interview.

Drawing on your own experience, can you write a description of what you feel in a situation such as this. Please note as many features as you can recall in the space provided.

Commentary

Here are some of the things you might have included:

- increased heart rate
- pounding heart
- dry mouth
- cold, clammy hands
- sweating
- need to go to the lavatory
- a sense of 'rising to the occasion'
- increased awareness.

This summarises some of the effects of adrenaline. Clearly, this hormone influences many parts of the body.

Most of us experience the effects of adrenaline from time to time, in a relatively minor way. But for some people the conditions which cause them may be prolonged.

ACTIVITY 63　　　　　ALLOW **10** MINUTES

Resource 8 contains a first-hand account, from a war correspondent, of how it feels to be subject to continued and intense fear-provoking stimuli. Please read this through now and make a note of anything which:

- you do not understand

- you find particularly interesting

- might apply to people receiving health care.

Commentary

We will be returning to this account later, so that you can check how your understanding has improved and consider how it may be applied to the provision of nursing care.

How adrenaline works

It is clear that the effects of adrenaline on the body are very widespread. How does it do it? A full account of the mechanism of its action is outside the scope of this course, but we will consider one way in which it acts on some of its targets to illustrate how hormones such as this affect individual cells.

Adrenaline released into the bloodstream circulates around the body and comes into contact with all types of cells. It is a small molecule, and therefore can leave the plasma and enter the intercellular fluid. When it encounters a cell with a particular structure on its surface it can combine, at that particular place. Having done this it triggers off the appropriate response in that particular cell.

It follows that only cells with these structures – **receptor sites** – on their outer surface can be influenced by adrenaline. In other words, such cells are the targets for this hormone.

There is more than one kind of adrenaline receptor, each causing the cell on which it is located to respond in a different way when adrenaline combines with the receptor. The type of receptor on the cells of the SA node in the heart is termed a **beta receptor**. There are similar receptors on the surfaces of the atrial and ventricular muscle cells. When adrenaline combines with these beta receptors it causes the heart muscles to become more receptive to stimuli and able to contract more rapidly. It can make the ventricular muscle so responsive that it throws off spontaneous contractions (**extrasystoles** or **ectopic beats**).

When describing the effects of fear and nervousness (Activity 62) you may have identified effects on your heart. People say things like 'My heart was hammering in my chest' or 'My heart missed a beat.' These are the effects of adrenaline, after it combines with the beta receptors. The author of Resource 8 describes the 'turbo-charged heart'.

People who are very nervous before a public appearance (such as musicians and actors) sometimes take drugs called beta blockers to help them stay calm. A **beta blocker** (such as propranolol) is a drug which binds to the beta receptor sites and prevents any naturally released adrenaline from docking there and increasing the heart rate.

Why is adrenaline produced?

You have seen that adrenaline is produced in response to emotional stimuli, such as anxiety and fear. It is also released from the adrenal medulla in response to other stimuli, including:

- cold

- low arterial blood pressure

- low blood sugar

- strenuous exercise.

This suggests that its function is to help the body to respond to these environmental challenges. From the work you have done in this unit you will perhaps deduce that the response will be part of the body's homeostatic mechanism and the result will be to maintain the constant internal environment.

ACTIVITY 64   ALLOW **10** MINUTES

Reflect on this list. Drawing upon your existing knowledge of physiology, can you work out what effect adrenaline might have on different parts of the body in order to bring about a response to these challenges?

Commentary

Table 8 shows some of the answers which you could have included. It includes a note of how adrenaline triggers these responses.

Stimuli which cause adrenaline production	Response	Reason for response
Exposure to cold	Increased heat production Reduced heat loss	Adrenaline speeds up the release and use of glucose. Adrenaline causes constriction of skin surface blood vessels.
Reduced arterial BP	Increased cardiac output Increased peripheral resistance	Adrenaline increases heart rate and stroke volume Adrenaline causes constriction of blood vessels in the skin and peripheral tissues.
Low blood sugar	Increased mobilisation of glucose from storage Reduced uptake of glucose by cells	Adrenaline speeds up the breakdown of glycogen (the glucose stores) and slows down the uptake of glucose into the cells.
Exercise	Increased blood flow to muscles	Adrenaline dilates blood vessels supplying muscles.

Table 8 Effects produced by adrenaline.

In all these cases, we can see adrenaline acting to restore the balance. Notice that its effects vary from place to place. For example, it causes constriction of skin surface blood vessels but dilation of vessels supplying voluntary muscles. It causes the response which is appropriate to the homeostatic need.

2: Adrenaline and the nervous system

Most of the reasons for adrenaline production which we have discussed are external stimuli – things that happen in the outside world. The body recognises that these things are happening and converts this information into action, including adrenaline release. Look again at the first paragraphs of Resource 8 to see a graphic description of how quickly it takes place. Let's consider how it happens.

The recognition of stimuli and the transmission of information are functions of the nervous system. The release of adrenaline provides a useful introduction to the way that messages travel around the nervous system and this will lead to the closing session of the unit in which we are going to consider pain.

The cells in the adrenal medulla which produce adrenaline are large cells, clumped around blood capillaries. They contain stores of adrenaline in granular structures (**chromaffin granules**). Each cell is supplied by a small branch of a sympathetic nerve (the **splanchnic** nerve) which terminates very close to the cell surface.

When a nerve impulse from the brain or spinal cord travels along this branch of the nerve it causes the release of a **neurotransmitter** at the nerve ending. This substance passes across the tiny space between the nerve end and the cell membrane and affects the membrane structure, causing calcium ions to flow into the cell.

The granules containing stored adrenaline are sensitive to the presence of calcium. When the amount of calcium is increased, the granules open and pour out their contents directly into the blood. This sequence is summarised in *Figure 17*.

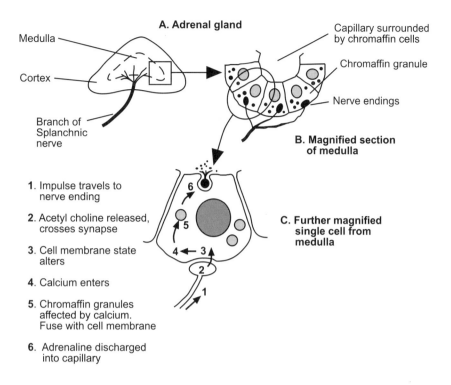

A. Adrenal gland

Medulla

Cortex

Capillary surrounded
by chromaffin cells

Chromaffin granule

Nerve endings

Branch of
Splanchnic
nerve

**B. Magnified section
of medulla**

1. Impulse travels to
nerve ending

2. Acetyl choline released,
crosses synapse

3. Cell membrane state
alters

4. Calcium enters

5. Chromaffin granules
affected by calcium.
Fuse with cell membrane

6. Adrenaline discharged
into capillary

**C. Further magnified
single cell from
medulla**

Figure 17 The discharge of adrenaline

The actual details of this process are outside the scope of this introductory course. However, we have included some of them here to illustrate the important idea that communication through the nervous system involves:

- changes in the state of cell membranes

- neurotransmitters, which make links between nerve endings and cells.

We'll be looking at these in more detail in the notes that follow.

The nerve impulse

Early on in this unit you looked at the membrane of a red blood cell from the point of view of its osmotic properties – allowing water but not other substances to pass. We said then that this was a very simplified view of cell membranes.

In fact, the complexity of these structures is astonishing. The way substances cross them is much more elaborate than we used to suppose. It's not just a question of having the right size 'holes' in the membrane to allow different things through. Rather, there are many different kinds of 'gates', each one allowing a particular substance through. One could liken this situation to a sports stadium with different turnstiles for ticket holders, home supporters, visitors and so on. To get into the stadium you need the right kind of ticket for your gate.

But the cellular 'stadium' is much more sophisticated. On the outside surface there are receptor zones which influence the gates in a variety of ways. They may open the gates, allowing substances to pass through, or they may alter the structure of the gate and influence the internal structure of the membrane.

When a nerve cell is stimulated at any point, its membrane is affected and some of the gates open, allowing sodium and potassium ions to move in and out. Before the gates open, the distribution of these ions (which, as you will remember, carry an electric charge) produces a specific charge across the membrane. When the gates open, the charge changes. This affects the adjacent section of membrane and causes gates to open there too, and so on, across the nerve cell and down to the nerve end. This is the **nerve impulse** – a self-generating wave of electrical activity which passes from the point of stimulation to the nerve ending. It all comes about through changes to the nerve cell membrane.

The structure of one kind of nerve cell is shown in *Figure 18*.

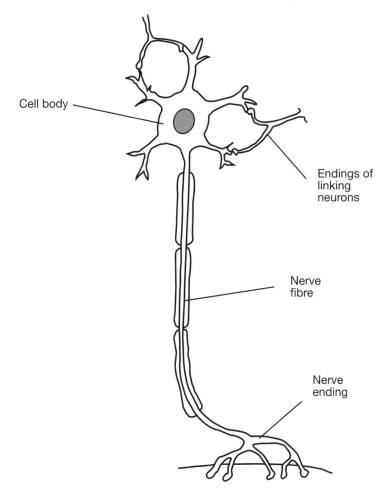

Cell body

Endings of linking neurons

Nerve fibre

Nerve ending

Figure 18 The structure of a neuron

This shows that the cell has an elaborate structure, consisting of the main section (cell body) and a number of spiky outgrowths. The cell body and all its spikes form a unit termed a **neuron**.

Neurons come in many different shapes, depending on their location and function. Some have many spikes and some just a few. These may be all similar in length or, as in the case of the example in *Figure 18*, one may be much longer than the others. This is the case where the spike, together with many others, forms a nerve, when it is termed a **nerve fibre**.

The spikes transmit information, in the form of nerve impulses, into or out from the cell body. Those which carry impulses away from their cells may end on the surface of another nerve cell or a cell in the tissue which they supply.

If it is to have any effect, the nerve impulse must pass across the tiny gap (the **synapse**) between the nerve end and the next cell. In other words, the changes which the nerve impulse causes in the membrane of the neuron must somehow be transmitted across that gap to the next neuron or other type of cell which it supplies.

Neurotransmitters

The nerve impulse is a form of electrical activity. The gap between the nerve end and the next cell is a fluid-filled space. The impulse cannot jump across this gap like a spark in an electrical circuit. It has to be converted into chemical activity in order to cross that space. This is where neurotransmitters come in. These chemicals are released when the electrical impulse reaches one side of a synapse. They pass across it and influence the membrane on the other side causing changes in that membrane which lead to the initiation of electrical activity there. So the impulse travels from one cell to the next.

You have already seen, however, that nerve fibres may end, not on another neuron, but upon a structure whose activity they control, such as the adrenal medulla. Neurotransmitters are produced here, too, altering the membrane of the target cell in some way and thus bringing about change. So throughout the nervous system and the structures it controls we have the same pattern recurring: electrical activity alternating with chemical activity. But what starts the whole sequence off?

To understand this, let's revisit Resource 8. Here the author describes the response to a fear-provoking stimulus – a loud noise. A noise is caused by disturbance of the air, in other words, by mechanical activity. (In this case the disturbance is caused by a firework, but the fear arises from the possibility that it is something more dangerous.) This mechanical effect is picked up by the ears, where nerve fibres ending in specialised receptors are situated. Here mechanical changes, rather than chemical changes, cause the generation of nerve impulses.

At the interface between the body and the outside world there are batteries of receptors – each specialised to respond to a different kind of environmental stimulus and turn it into nerve impulses. They include sound receptors, light receptors, chemical receptors, pressure receptors, and so on. Although their structures are different they all have the same effect – to convert stimuli into patterns of nerve impulses which carry information to the brain.

The internal state of the body is also monitored by receptors. You have come across osmoreceptors and stretch receptors. They also respond to stimuli and, through their specialised structures, convert these into nerve impulses. So we can begin to put together a picture of the activity of the nervous system in these terms:

1 stimulus
2 receptors
3 electrical transmission (nerve impulse)   (3 and 4 may be
4 chemical transmission (e.g. neurotransmitters)   repeated
5 end result.   several times)

Although many of the pathways through the nervous system are extremely complex, they are all based on this pattern. The end product can be many things, including the production of hormones. Let's consider an example, of the relationship between nerves and hormone production in more detail.

Under stress, the hypothalamus receives nerve impulses from the conscious parts of the brain. Neurons in the hypothalamus release chemicals which pass directly to the pituitary gland and cause this to release several different hormones (including the TSH, which you have already met, and ACTH: adreno-corticotrophic hormone). These, in turn, act on other endocrine glands, like the thyroid, to stimulate the appropriate response.

At the same time, the stressful stimuli trigger off other sequences of nervous and hormonal activity. These include impulses in the sympathetic nervous system which result in the production of neurotransmitters whose effects add to those we have just described. One of these is **noradrenaline**, a substance similar to adrenaline which acts as a neurotransmitter and also acts to increase the blood supply to the heart muscle.

So the total response to fear consists of a number of separate pathways, each adding to what the author of Resource 8 terms 'the body's potent survival chemistry'.

ACTIVITY 65   ALLOW 10 MINUTES

Re-read the first two paragraphs of Resource 8, and referring to the sections you have just read, make a note of how two of the chemicals mentioned come to be produced.

Commentary

The chemicals you will recognise are adrenaline and noradrenaline.

- Adrenaline is released from the adrenal gland, in response to stimulation by the sympathetic nervous system
- Noradrenaline is released by the sympathetic nervous system.

What we have just described is part of the body's 'fight or flight' response, which happens automatically when a person is faced with real danger, or a situation which is thought to be dangerous.

The next activity invites you to put all this together by thinking through what happens in a practical situation.

ACTIVITY 66

ALLOW 10 MINUTES

Imagine that you are involved in the care of a person with a mental health problem which, from time to time, changes his perception of reality. During one of these episodes, as you and your colleague approach to ask if he will come for lunch, he cries out in fear 'Get away from me, don't hurt me'. You realise that he sees you as two very threatening figures. His 'fight or flight' system is in full operation. Suggest the changes that this will bring about in the following parts of his body:

1 eyes

2 heart

3 blood supply to intestines

4 blood supply to muscles of arms and legs

5 blood glucose levels

6 lungs

7 blood supply to the skin.

Commentary

1 The pupils are dilated, allowing more light into the eyes.

2 The heart-rate is increased and the pumping action of the heart is increased so that more blood is pumped out of the heart for each beat, i.e. the stroke volume is increased.

3 The intestinal blood supply is reduced, as this organ is not vital in a stressful situation. This may eventually lead to nausea and vomiting.

4 The muscles of the arms and legs are vital in frightening and stressful situations. Blood vessels to these tissues are dilated by adrenaline so that the muscles receive more nutrition and oxygen to cope with the extra work.

5 Adrenaline causes breakdown of glycogen to glucose in the liver. The glucose then flows into the bloodstream, where it is available for energy needs.

6 In a stressful situation the body requires more oxygen to burn up (metabolise) extra glucose from the liver. Adrenaline causes relaxation of the muscle of the bronchioles and so more oxygen can be breathed in.

7   The blood supply to the skin is not vital in a frightening situation and the body must preserve its heat. Noradrenaline constricts the blood vessels in the skin and some of this blood is redirected to areas where it is needed urgently such as the muscles (see 4 above). The skin of a frightened person may therefore appear cool and pale.

You would probably be able to recognise some of these effects of fear in this person, and it would be important to take steps to reduce, not escalate, his fear and to recognise the source of any aggressive behaviour that accompanied it.

Under normal circumstances, the response to fear or stress is relatively short-lived, and feedback systems bring the levels of hormones and neurotransmitters back to normal. However, prolonged and continued stress of this kind means a prolonged disturbance of body chemistry. In Resource 8 the author suggests that severely altered behaviour may result. You might like to discuss this with your colleagues and consider situations in which people receiving care are subject to prolonged exposure to fear-inducing situations.

We are normally unaware of the constant activity of electrical and chemical transmission occurring throughout our bodies. Only when things go wrong in some way do we become conscious of the process. We then experience sensations of discomfort or pain. We are going to conclude this unit by focusing on this very important aspect of nursing care – understanding the person who has pain.

3: Experiencing pain

Pain is often the first indication of disease or trauma. It is a very private experience. No one can appreciate or measure another person's pain. It is clear that what a person actually experiences is due to many factors beside the strength and character of the painful stimulus. However, some of the underlying physiology of pain is well described and by drawing on this information nurses can do a great deal to assist the person who is in pain. Let's begin to explore this by thinking about the kind of pain which we commonly experience in normal life.

Everyday pain

The sensation of pain is started by receptors which detect various kinds of tissue damage, or rather, the products of tissue damage or malfunction.

ACTIVITY 67   ALLOW 10 MINUTES

Drawing on your own experience, can you identify some different kinds of pain that you have experienced in the past? For each one, suggest the kind of tissue damage or malfunction that was producing the sensation of pain. Aim to suggest five or six examples.

Commentary

Table 9 lists some common causes of 'everyday' pain. These are things that many people have experienced at some time.

Skin cuts and scratches	Damage to skin and underlying tissue
Nettle stings	Poison injected into skin
Surface burn	Destruction of skin and underlying tissue
Headache	Increased pressure
Abdominal pain from digestive upset	Strong muscular contractions
Ankle or wrist sprain	Damage to tissues of joint
Painful stiffness after exercise	Trauma to muscle following over-exertion

Table 9 Common causes of 'everyday' pain

These everyday occurrences all arise because of tissue damage, inflammation or inadequate blood supply to muscle.

Nerve impulses in pain

The receptors which pick up the painful stimuli are at the end of nerve fibres which carry impulses to the **central nervous system (CNS)**. These fibres belong to **sensory** neurons in the brain and spinal cord – nerve cells which receive incoming impulses and transmit them on the other parts of the CNS.

Each sensory neuron connects, via synapses, with neurons in the CNS (as shown in *Figure 19*). The incoming impulses may then be sent along a chain of neurons to the parts of the brain which produce conscious sensation.

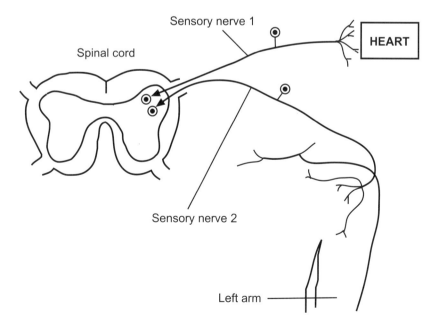

Figure 19 Sensory neurons

Nerve fibres are of different types. Some conduct impulses faster than others. For example, some fibres are surrounded by sheaths of a fatty material (**myelin**) which is a little like an insulator on an electric cable. This sheath has gaps along its length and the nerve impulse moves quickly from one gap to the next, giving a faster rate of conduction than fibres which do not have the sheath (unmyelinated fibres).

Pain in the skin or superficial parts of the body is usually detected by receptors attached to myelinated fibres. It tends to be sharp, whereas pain in the internal organs is more likely to be conducted along unmyelinated fibres and be dull or aching in character.

ACTIVITY 68   ALLOW 2 MINUTES

Thinking again about your own experience of these two types of pain in everyday life, what kind of response do you make to them?

Commentary

We usually flinch or draw back from a sharp, surface kind of pain, even a pin prick. This is the typical reaction of a person having sutures removed: it takes a lot of willpower to keep still.

On the other hand, we usually 'guard' a deep, aching pain – by keeping still, holding the affected area or perhaps applying gentle warmth.

Referred pain

Activity 68 raises the question of whether we always protect the right place. One of the authors vividly remembers having severe toothache, going to the dentist, and having an upper molar extracted. The dentist looked puzzled. When the anaesthetic wore off the pain returned in full force in the corresponding lower molar. The abscess was in the lower jaw, but the pain was 'referred' to the upper.

This phenomenon happens when the sensory fibres from two areas are close together in the spinal cord. The brain misinterprets the source of the pain.

ACTIVITY 69   ALLOW 5 MINUTES

Please refer back to *Figure 19* which shows the two sensory pathways involved in Mr Granville's experience of a heart attack. Check back on his symptoms and see if you can explain the location of his pain.

Commentary

Mr Granville experienced his pain in his left shoulder and neck. Sensory nerve 2 has its origin in the spinal cord close to sensory nerve 1, from the heart. So lack of oxygen and damage to the heart muscle caused referred pain in the shoulder area.

Pain pathways

Suppose that you bang your shin on a low table – a very painful experience. Your instinct is probably to rub it hard. Have you ever wondered why that should be the automatic response?

To explain this common phenomenon we need to look at the pathways taken by nerve impulses produced by painful stimuli as they travel to the CNS.

Let's concentrate on the pain-conducting fibres attached to the receptors responding to a blow on the shin. These form part of a nerve arising from the spinal cord (a spinal nerve). As in all nerves, many fibres travel together, conveying impulses to cell bodies in the spinal cord.

When the impulses caused by the painful stimulus reach the spinal cord they are transmitted across synapses to other neurons which carry the impulses upwards to the brain.

However, lots of other non-painful impulses are transmitted along the same route at the same time. The neurons which they reach may modify the signals in the pain-conducting fibres and may stop them from reaching the brain and producing conscious sensation. This mechanism is termed the **spinal gates**. The stimuli from the pain receptors will only get through the gates if there are relatively few non-painful impulses in comparison to the numbers of pain impulses.

Rubbing the area close to the site of a painful stimulus sends large numbers of non-painful impulses up to the spinal gates and may succeed in preventing any sensation of pain.

However, this is not the end of the story. There are other pathways in the nervous system which affect the way that pain is experienced by the conscious brain, as the next activity reminds us.

ACTIVITY 70 ALLOW **10** MINUTES

Drawing on your own observation of the way people respond to pain, make a list of some of the factors which, in your opinion, might affect the response to a potentially painful stimulus.

Commentary

Some of the factors you might have suggested include:

Cultural and social influences: What response to pain is permissible in a particular family or culture? How is the child's experience of pain handled within the family?

Personality: How self-contained or expressive is the person?

Anxiety: This may produce a vicious circle in which anxiety enhances pain and thus creates more anxiety, and so on.

Anticipation: Waiting for something to happen may heighten the experience of pain, for example, if a person knows for some time that they are about to undergo a painful procedure.

Past experience: People who have experienced pain, especially severe pain, in the past often find that they judge present pain in comparison to their previous sensation.

Stressful, emotional or exciting situations: These may heighten or reduce pain sensation, e.g.:

- a footballer may have a serious injury but not begin to feel exceptional pain until the excitement of the game is over
- a soldier may be in severe pain on the battlefield but the pain lessens when he is moved to the calmer atmosphere of a hospital area

Distraction: Pain may sometimes be reduced by relieving boredom and encouraging pastimes.

Some of these factors show that the conscious brain can exert an influence over the experience of pain. This is because there are nerve pathways from the brain (the **descending inhibitory pathways**) which transmit impulses down from the brain and modify the pain signals which are travelling up towards the brain.

So many features of a person's past and present experience are brought to bear on the experience of pain and the response that is made to pain. It is important for nurses to be aware of the individual nature of this response, so that they can understand what the person in pain is telling them.

Neurotransmitters in pain perception

As we are all aware, pain is not a simple thing. Its quality and our response to it are both very varied. So it is not surprising to find that the pathways through which pain is sensed are very complex, involving many different neurotransmitters. It is not clear why there should be so many, or what part they all play.

However, we do know that there are some substances which block the action of these pain-producing transmitters. Morphine, for example, acts by binding onto the surface of cells which respond to signals coming from pain receptors. This prevents them from producing the chemicals needed to send the pain stimulus forward. Morphine is a very powerful **analgesic** and has just the right structure to combine with specific receptor sites on these cells.

These **opioid receptors** are not there for the purpose of 'receiving' morphine, since this is not a substance which naturally occurs in the human body. They are the sites at which the body's natural analgesics exert their action in the descending inhibitory pathways described above. These substances were originally called 'endogenous morphines', a term which has now been abbreviated to **endorphins**. They are produced in response to exercise and stressful stimuli, ready to protect the body from the immediate consequences of injury.

The effects of pain

The ability to recognise that a person is experiencing pain is very important for nurses. It is useful to distinguish between acute and chronic pain here.

Acute pain is usually due to an event, such as surgery or trauma, and has a sudden onset. So the person may have received a very frightening stimulus and be in a state of shock. The effects of the fight or flight system are apparent, for example, pallor, sweating, rapid pulse and dilated pupils.

If the acute pain is severe and prolonged, more extreme manifestation of shock may follow – for example, vomiting or fainting.

The person's behavioural response will depend on the severity of the pain and their natural way of reacting to it. People in acute pain may express themselves forcibly or may be very still and quiet.

Chronic pain may last for months or longer. It may have a more gradual onset. Normal sleep patterns may be disturbed, and the person feels there is no prospect of the pain ending. These longer-term effects often add depression to the continued physiological response to pain, with consequences for the person's whole lifestyle.

Managing pain

From this brief outline of the physiology and effects of pain it should be clear that managing pain involves both pain relief and other types of support. This is another area where the clinical nurse specialist has an important role – particularly in the management of patients with pain during the closing stages of their lives. Here a knowledge of the underlying physiology is needed to understand the action and side effects of analgesics, the response of the body to pain and the recognition of the person's experience.

This is a very large subject, outside the scope of this introductory course, but the section which follows will give you the opportunity to apply what you have already learnt in this area.

First, read Resource 9, which provides some extended background information to help with the next activity.

ACTIVITY 71 — ALLOW 5 MINUTES

Once again, drawing on your own experience, can you think of an occasion when you were unaware that you had hurt yourself until some time after the event?

If you can, describe what happened, and see if you can provide a physiological explanation. (Use a separate sheet of paper if you need to.)

Commentary

Here is a short story told by a nurse who tried this activity.

'I can remember having a slight accident in my car. It was a side impact and I was thrown against the offside door. My three-year-old daughter was in the back seat, strapped in. It wasn't until I'd got her out, checked her over and got someone to take care of her that I realised my shoulder was hurting like hell. I had a broken collar bone.' A possible explanation here is that non-painful impulses were closing the spinal gates and preventing this person from experiencing pain at this time. However, this seems rather unlikely – after she has been knocked about in the accident more painful than non-painful impulses are likely to be travelling up to her brain.

Clearly, in this case her conscious brain was suppressing the painful stimuli from her damaged shoulder until she had satisfied her overpowering urge to protect her child. Something other than the pain gates must have been responsible for this.

This is an example of the operation of the descending inhibitory pathways which interact with the pain-sensitive neurons near the spinal gates.

People in pain

Let us conclude this session by looking at some examples of people experiencing pain and using their stories to draw together all the things you have studied in this unit. This will show how nurses who have a good understanding of physiological principles can assist the people they care for.

We suggest you read all the case studies first and then carry out the activities at the end of each one.

Case Study 1: a minor injury

David, an eight-year-old boy, was playing in his back garden with his friend Mahayed on a hot August day. They brought out glasses of orange juice but soon wished they hadn't, because several wasps started to take an interest. David suddenly screamed in pain and fear. A wasp, crawling on the rim of his glass, had stung him on the lip. He dropped his glass and ran indoors, with his hands clasped to his mouth.

David's mum put a cold cloth on the bite and found that rubbing the skin of his cheek helped relieve the pain. She didn't make a lot of fuss, but was a bit worried as she saw his face starting to swell and took him to the GP.

The practice nurse saw him in reception and brought him straight through to be seen. She checked inside his mouth very carefully and asked David if he had any other stings, beside the one on his lip. David was sure that he had spat the wasp out quickly and that it had only stung his lip.

An hour later, David was back home, still complaining about his sore lip but otherwise showing no ill effects. Mahayed came round and David suddenly felt well enough to rush out to play.

Follow-up questions:

1 When David ran inside, what signs of shock would his mother notice?

2 How can you explain the pain and swelling which David experienced?

3 In what way did his mother's instinctive response alleviate his pain?

4   Why was the practice nurse so careful to check for other stings?

5   How do you think this experience will affect David's future view of stinging insects?

6   How similar is David's experience to that of a young child being given an injection?

Case Study 2: the executive

Edward Gregory is a 54-year-old bank manager who is overweight and smokes 20 cigarettes a day. His doctor has explained that these problems may affect his heart but he finds difficulty changing his lifestyle. In his office one day Edward experiences a severe crushing pain in his chest that radiates to his jaw and along his left arm. He has several friends who have had heart attacks, is aware of the symptoms, and is very frightened. He manages to summon his secretary and she finds him slumped on his desk, very pale and sweaty. She telephones an ambulance and he is taken to hospital.

In hospital, Edward is interviewed by a doctor. She reassures him that his pain will be treated promptly. This in itself appears to alleviate his pain somewhat and his normal colour returns. He is given an injection of diamorphine (heroin) to relieve the pain and is prescribed regular doses of this drug together with some oxygen. However, the nurses notice that he is sleeping and do not give any more diamorphine until he complains of pain and is visibly frightened.

Follow-up questions

1   What non-physiological events may have contributed to Edward's experience of pain?

2   Why did he get pain in his jaw and left arm?

3   Which part of the nervous system is responsible for Edward becoming pale and clammy and which hormone is involved?

4   What type of damage to the heart muscle do you feel is responsible for the pain that he is suffering?

5   What part of his care may have activated the descending inhibitory pathways?

6   Why are the nurses reluctant to give further diamorphine?

If possible, discuss with your colleagues how you think Edward's pain should be managed.

Case Study 3: a familiar nursing story

Shirley Chan is 43 years old and has been nursing for 20 years. Two years ago she hurt her back while lifting a patient. She was told she had trapped a nerve and the tissues were inflamed. Bed rest was advised, together with anti-inflammatory drugs. This was unsuccessful. Shirley was admitted to hospital and traction was applied for two weeks to try to ease the trapped nerve. She became very depressed and irritable and the pain became the main focus of her life. She seemed to require increasing quantities of drugs. Dihydrocodeine was prescribed, one of the opioid group of drugs, but this simply made Shirley very disorientated and constipated. She spent many sleepless nights. The nurses obtained a video recorder for her use and she seemed to be better while watching her favourite programmes which her partner brought in. Finally she admitted she could see no end in sight to her suffering and the consultant referred her to the pain control team.

Firstly the opioid drugs were slowly withdrawn and a weak electrical stimulator was applied to an area near the site of Shirley's pain. Shirley held the control button for this and for the first time seemed to gain some control over her pain. A course of hypnotherapy helped Shirley to take a more positive view of controlling her pain and a course of amitriptyline, an antidepressant drug that increases the levels of noradrenaline, proved enough to get Shirley home and back in control of her life.

Follow-up questions

1   At what stage do you think acute pain becomes chronic in type?

2   What part of the pain-relieving pathway would hypnotherapy and noradrenaline help to activate?

If possible, discuss with your colleagues any other types of illness causing chronic pain.

Answers to Case Study questions

Case Study 1

1   David would probably look pale and wide-eyed and his mother might notice his heart beating rapidly.

2   The release of histamine, caused by the wasp sting, causes pain by stimulating pain receptors, and localised oedema as part of the triple response.

3   Rubbing David's cheek near to the sting provides counter-irritation which helps to close the spinal gate by producing more neurotransmitters in the spinal cord that inhibit the pain signals.

    Using a cold compress may provide a numbing sensation at the point of the sting. It may also cause vasoconstriction in the local tissues and help to reduce the spread of the stinging chemicals.

4   If the wasp had stung David inside his mouth the tissue oedema produced might have caused respiratory obstruction.

5   David will associate these insects with pain and may well avoid them. His fear and anticipation may affect his experience of pain if he is stung again.

6   There are many similarities between the two situations:

    ● lack of understanding
    ● fear and shock
    ● acute pain
    ● withdrawal response
    ● establishment of fearful anticipation
    ● relief of distress by distraction.

Case Study 2

1 Edward has already been told by his doctor that his sedentary job and his heavy smoking may cause heart problems, so he has a good idea what is happening when he gets chest pain.

Several of his friends have already had heart attacks so that he can anticipate what is going to happen to him and the pain he is likely to get.

All these previous experiences probably inhibit the descending inhibitory centres and magnify his experience of pain.

2 This is referred pain. It arises because sensory fibres from the left arm and jaw join the spinal cord close to the sensory fibres from the heart. The pain from the ischaemic heart muscle is therefore sensed to be coming from these two areas as well as from the chest.

3 Edward is very frightened, and therefore his sympathetic nervous system is activated. The production of both noradrenaline and adrenaline will increase to produce a pale, clammy skin, together with increased heart rate. The effect of adrenaline on the heart following a heart attack can be so powerful that extra heart beats (ectopic beats) can be produced, so causing a peculiar heart rhythm (arrhythmia). This can be very dangerous in the early period after a heart attack.

4 A heart attack is usually caused by a blockage of one or more of the coronary arteries. Initially this deprives the heart muscle of oxygen and allows a build-up of chemicals, which produce pain. This is the pain of angina. If the blockage of the artery cannot be by-passed then that small piece of muscle is starved of oxygen and will die. This produces continuous pain and releases chemicals from the dying cells, which causes further pain. The size and position of the infarcted muscle determines whether his heart can recover and function again.

5 The reassurance from the medical and nursing staff will to some extent counteract Edward's previous knowledge and anticipation of these events and so activate the descending inhibitory centres.

6 Diamorphine is a very powerful drug and because of its habit-forming properties (addiction) its use is very strictly controlled. Like all other opioids, it has side effects. The most relevant for the nursing staff are that it depresses respiration and causes sedation with a feeling of wellbeing. The latter effect is very useful after a heart attack but if Edward suffers respiratory depression he may not breathe deeply enough or at an adequate rate to get sufficient oxygen.

Case Study 3

1 It is sometimes very difficult to decide when acute pain becomes chronic in nature, especially if you are the person suffering the pain. Chronic pain may last for months or longer and ultimately cause depression. The distinction between acute and chronic pain is made because certain treatments and drugs work better on one kind of pain than on the other, or may be more appropriate to one type of pain.

2   Hypnotherapy has several actions on pain perception:

- it tends to have a calming influence

- it can be used as a distraction treatment so that priorities are focused away from the pain and the patient concentrates attention/energy on some other aspect of life

- the patient may be able to achieve some degree of pain control by taking a positive attitude.

All these suggest a central influence and it is likely that the descending inhibitory pathways are activated during hypnotherapy.

Noradrenaline is actually present in one of the descending inhibitory pathways as a neurotransmitter. In this pathway excess noradrenaline production leads to a decrease in pain perception.

Using these case studies should have shown you that pain is all around us, whether a child playing in the garden bumps a knee or someone has a major heart attack. It is important to understand how we sense pain and ultimately how that sensation may be modified by both spinal gates and the descending inhibitory pathways. You have seen how pain may be referred to different parts of the body that may well not be involved with the original pain sensation.

You have looked at some of the variety of substances that can act as neurotransmitters to convey pain impulses to the brain, and you have seen that the consequences of pain are very complicated. However, despite this complexity it is possible, with a little appreciation of basic physiology, to understand what is happening to a person who is in pain or whose systems are out of balance as a result of illness, stress or trauma.

A final look at Resource 8 will reinforce this point.

ACTIVITY 72   ALLOW 15 MINUTES

Read through Resource 8 once more. Turn back to Activity 63 where you noted down things that you did not understand. Check these to see if you can now explain all the points that are raised in this piece of work. Here is a checklist of the main points:

1   How hormones and neurotransmitters are produced after a fear-provoking stimulus (paragraphs 1 and 2).

2   How the body responds in a fight or flight situation (paragraphs 3 to 6).

3   Why long-term stress may cause cardiovascular disease and kidney failure (paragraph 15).

4   How homeostatic systems may be 'reset' in response to abnormal conditions (paragraph 16).

Commentary

If you are satisfied that your understanding of these topics has improved and you can apply this understanding to patient care you have achieved the main objectives of this unit.

Perhaps we could conclude by considering the stress to which people receiving health care are subject.

ACTIVITY 73   ALLOW **30 MINUTES**

Up to 20 minutes in discussion, 10 minutes on your own

Working alone or with a group of colleagues, compile a list of situations in which patients or clients are likely to be subject to long- or short-term stress (arising from fear or pain). Then select one of them and discuss:

- the likely effects of the stress experienced on that person
- the role of the nurse in assisting that person.

Commentary

You will have made your own selection, which may be different from ours. Here are some suggestions. There are many more:

- waiting in an outpatient clinic
- being on a waiting list for surgery
- waiting for anticipated bad news
- getting ready to go home after a long admission to hospital
- managing at home with a painful, chronic condition
- having had an operation cancelled
- recovering after surgery.

People in all these situations will exhibit some of the things you have been considering in Session Six. We hope that you can now apply your knowledge of physiology to plan care in any of these cases.

Summary of Session Six

- Adrenaline is part of the body's response to stress of many kinds.

- Its effects prepare the body for 'fight or flight'.

- Nerve impulses travel by means of both electrical and chemical transmission.

- Pain is a very individual experience.

- Many factors influence a person's perception of pain.

- Nurses need to be able to recognise fear and pain and to understand the physiology of the body's response to short- and long-term exposure to these stresses.

LEARNING REVIEW

Now that you have completed your work on this unit, you may like to assess your progress and understanding. You can do this by completing the following learning review, and comparing your answers with those that you gave before you started Session One.

	Not at all	Partly	Quite well	Very well

Session One
I can:
- explain, in general terms, the relevance of physiological principles to the delivery of nursing care

	☐	☐	☐	☐
describe the volume and distribution of fluid in the human body	☐	☐	☐	☐
explain the idea of water balance	☐	☐	☐	☐
outline the function of intercellular fluid in providing a stable internal environment	☐	☐	☐	☐
describe the effects of fluid deprivation on the human body	☐	☐	☐	☐
define the term 'oedema'	☐	☐	☐	☐
describe the forces which result in the formation of intercellular fluid	☐	☐	☐	☐
explain the consequences of an imbalance in these forces	☐	☐	☐	☐
predict what will happen if any one of these forces, for example, the osmotic pressure of the plasma, changes drastically	☐	☐	☐	☐
define the term homeostasis and understand what it means in relation to the body's fluid balance	☐	☐	☐	☐
outline the principles underlying the nursing care of a person with peripheral oedema.	☐	☐	☐	☐

Session Two
I can:

	Not at all	Partly	Quite well	Very well
outline the structure of the normal kidney and the way in which urine is produced	☐	☐	☐	☐
explain the effects of reduced fluid intake	☐	☐	☐	☐
explain why fluids are given, as a matter of urgency, to casualties who have suffered blood loss	☐	☐	☐	☐
describe the role of the kidney in the homeostatic processes which regulate BP	☐	☐	☐	☐
explain the principle of feedback control as it applies to the renin/angiotensin system	☐	☐	☐	☐

	Not at all	Partly	Quite well	Very well
• describe and explain the symptoms of chronic and acute renal failure	☐	☐	☐	☐
• discuss the role of the clinical nurse specialist working in a renal unit	☐	☐	☐	☐
• outline the relationship between renal and cardiac function.	☐	☐	☐	☐

Session Three

I can:

	Not at all	Partly	Quite well	Very well
• describe, in outline, the structure and function of the heart	☐	☐	☐	☐
• identify the way in which blood flows through the heart to the lungs and the rest of the body	☐	☐	☐	☐
• explain the way that the heart beat is initiated and apply this understanding to supporting patients undergoing electrocardiogram investigations	☐	☐	☐	☐
• describe how the heart rate is varied to meet the changing needs of the body	☐	☐	☐	☐
• explain how variations in the heart beat contribute to the maintenance of homeostasis	☐	☐	☐	☐
• explain the relationship between the activity of the heart and the blood pressure	☐	☐	☐	☐
• identify the effects of right- and left-sided heart failure	☐	☐	☐	☐
• explain how oedema may be caused by heart failure	☐	☐	☐	☐
• outline the relationship between the cardiovascular and respiratory systems.	☐	☐	☐	☐

Session Four

I can:

	Not at all	Partly	Quite well	Very well
• describe what happens during normal breathing, including the respiratory movements and the exchange of gases at the lung surface	☐	☐	☐	☐
• explain the effects of breathing difficulty, in general terms	☐	☐	☐	☐
• outline the structure and characteristics of the lungs	☐	☐	☐	☐
• describe how the rate of breathing is controlled	☐	☐	☐	☐
• understand the effects of lung damage on the pulmonary and systemic circulation	☐	☐	☐	☐
• give an account, in outline only, of the role of histamine in the normal response to damage and in anaphylaxis	☐	☐	☐	☐
• discuss the nature of asthma and its effects on people	☐	☐	☐	☐
• use my understanding of physiology to suggest how nurses can best support people with asthma and other breathing problems.	☐	☐	☐	☐

	Not at all	Partly	Quite well	Very well

Session Five

I can:

- describe the role of the thyroid hormones in the control of temperature | ☐ | ☐ | ☐ | ☐
- discuss the contribution of the nervous and hormonal systems to the maintenance of temperature homeostasis | ☐ | ☐ | ☐ | ☐
- explain how heatstroke, pyrexia and hypothermia are brought about | ☐ | ☐ | ☐ | ☐
- outline the regular manner in which body temperature varies during the day | ☐ | ☐ | ☐ | ☐
- apply my knowledge of variations in body temperature to the provision of care. | ☐ | ☐ | ☐ | ☐

Session Six

I can:

- describe how adrenaline is produced and affects several body systems | ☐ | ☐ | ☐ | ☐
- outline the relationship between adrenaline and the sympathetic nervous system | ☐ | ☐ | ☐ | ☐
- explain how a nerve impulse travels along a nerve fibre | ☐ | ☐ | ☐ | ☐
- outline how neurotransmitters work
- draw a simple diagram of a neuron | ☐ | ☐ | ☐ | ☐
- recognise the signs which show that a person is afraid
- identify the causes of 'everyday' pain | ☐ | ☐ | ☐ | ☐
- describe how referred pain is caused | ☐ | ☐ | ☐ | ☐
- explain how painful stimuli can be modified in the nervous system | ☐ | ☐ | ☐ | ☐
- outline the role of the nurse in caring for people suffering from acute and chronic pain | ☐ | ☐ | ☐ | ☐
- relate the possible consequences of prolonged stress to patient care. | ☐ | ☐ | ☐ | ☐

RESOURCES SECTION

Contents

RESOURCE 1

Rowan Worsman,
Nursing Times,
October 19,
Vol 84, No 42, 1988

Haemodialysis: a fragile lifeline

Michael long outlived the eight months staff gave him when he was diagnosed with renal failure. Rowan Worsman describes how the quality of Michael's life deteriorated as he faced the problems of long-term dialysis.

Michael had a good job as a technician in a university research department.

This entailed many long distance business trips in England and abroad and, until his illness, he greatly enjoyed his work.

The family had always been used to going away a lot and enjoying many activities together. Michael had a great interest in his car and in their riverside home, Ivy Cottage. Along with their home went a stretch of river bank, and eventually they had to sell and live in a bungalow.

His wife Nora, who could not drive, worked full time for a blood bank but she had to give up her job for part-time work in order to look after Michael. She later developed heart problems caused by stress. Nora found it very difficult to accept their changing way of life, which meant staying at home more and seeing jobs in the house not being done.

Michael's illness first became apparent when he and his family were on holiday in Malta. He complained of feeling nauseated and tired. The rest of the family went off on their own as he felt unable to walk far. They thought he was just being a 'spoil-sport'. His condition did not improve on returning home. He saw his GP in November 1979, complaining of feeling generally unwell, tiredness, nausea and vomiting and breathlessness. He was unable to stand or walk for long, had headaches, lack of taste and deteriorating eyesight. His GP found Michael had quite marked hypertension.

In March 1980, Michael was admitted to hospital with malignant hypertension and left ventricular failure. A renal biopsy confirmed renal failure and, unknown to Michael and his family, the opinion was he had about eight months to live. There are no facilities in the hospital to which he was admitted for patients with renal failure; no haemodialysis or renal consultant. The consultant treating him referred him to the Manchester renal unit, partly because of his age and partly because of pressure from his family.

He began peritoneal dialysis and had a fistula formation in his arm for haemodialysis at a later stage. He remained in hospital many weeks until be became stable on peritoneal dialysis when he was allowed home for weekends, though he could not manage without some form of renal replacement.

Michael had his first haemodialysis in June 1980. His blood pressure was hard to control and captopril, which was then a new anti-hypertensive drug, was begun. He lost muscle weight and was off work for many months.

While he was feeling ill, he had to learn about his strict diet with protein, potassium and salt restriction and limited fluid allowance. He had to learn about his haemodialysis treatment, and to insert needles into his arm for dialysis; one of the most difficult aspects of treatment.

Nora had to rely on lifts to Manchester to see him, a journey of about 80 miles each way, and difficult to make by public transport. Little information was given to her by medical staff and she felt bewildered, with many unanswered questions. She also had most of the work and sorting out to do when it came to moving house later, an event which upset both of them, as they had planned to retire in Ivy Cottage.

The home dialysis administrator did go to see Nora and this proved very helpful. Unfortunately the home administrator changed jobs. The back-up help was not as good after this.

Haemodialysis was a whole new concept of living and thinking for Michael and his family. He had to learn to set up the dialysis machines, put himself on dialysis, dialyse and take himself off. He had to learn to deal with problems which could arise when on his own. A number of tests had to be passed satisfactorily during his dialysis training before he was allowed to dialyse at home. While training, he lived at home but spent three days a week going to Manchester to dialyse for eight hours. He often left home about 7am and returned about 9pm. During this time he still felt unwell, having great problems in controlling his blood pressure. The captopril began to have side-effects and he suffered with wind and vomiting. He wanted to return to work, as he feared losing his employment and financial stability.

Many arguments arose at home as Michael felt too tired to do or even want to do anything. His wife found this very hard to understand saying that haemodialysis gave quantity of life but not quality. He felt nauseated and vomited every day due to fluid restriction, the diet and his medication. He had to undergo tests to assess his degree of renal failure, which ruled out any chance of a kidney transplant. His severe hypertension would have destroyed a new kidney. The family were upset, thinking at first that he was refused a transplant because of his age.

A year later, by mid-1981, Michael looked much improved though he had lost a lot of weight. He was able to work two days a week and was quite happy.

He moved to a satellite dialysis unit 30 miles from his home, where there were no renal nurses, but patients could telephone the Manchester unit if they needed help. He changed his routine to dialysis for 10 hours twice a week. This he soon found too tiring. He also started to work for four days a week. He still had problems with nausea and vomiting and blood pressure control. His condition began to deteriorate.

The 10 hours twice weekly dialysis proved too much for him, and he became unwell. He refrained from saying anything to the medical staff, because he knew he would have to go back to dialysing eight hours three times a week, which may have meant losing his job. His condition deteriorated quickly two days after moving house. As he arrived at work he developed severe breathlessness and chest pain. He was taken home and then admitted to a Manchester hospital, where he remained for a week, with pneumonia.

After this episode he was back to dialysing for eight hours three times a week. A mass showed in his lungs on X-ray, and a month later cancer of the lung was diagnosed.

He was not told about the cancer until he and his wife had had their two weeks holiday in Blackpool. Neither he nor his family had any doubts about going ahead with the treatment offered. He was readmitted to Manchester where a thoracotomy and partial left lobectomy were performed.

He recovered well from this operation and the cancer had been cleared. Plans then went ahead to get him home and he had his first home haemodialysis just a month later.

There are a few holiday dialysis centres in England, so Michael and his wife took a holiday in the south. They stayed in a caravan, so he used a portable haemodialysis machine. He had training in the renal unit before he went, but while dialysing he became very ill. He had mistakenly dialysed for 2½ hours against water, instead of water and dialysate fluid. He got over this, although it did spoil their holiday. On returning home he had a blood transfusion and continued to dialyse at home. He was now working five days a week and dialysing three nights a week.

In mid-1984 he took a holiday in France with his family, near a dialysis centre. He had been complaining of midchest pain for six months, but nothing had been done about the condition. The pain increased during the summer and autumn, and he suffered a mild myocardial infarction in November, while at work. His condition worsened and in mid-June 1985 he was again admitted to Manchester. This time he underwent a triple cardiac by-pass operation, using grafts from his legs. He soon recovered, although he did suffer a pulmonary embolus just after going home. This meant a few more days in hospital, but in the end he recovered very well.

He had arranged financial support for his wife as he accepted that he would not live for very long on haemodialysis, and once said 'he could never imagine a man of 60, needling himself'.

He retired from work at the end of 1985. He had dropped a lot of his hobbies from the beginning of his illness. He feared losing touch and slowing down; to him retirement was the end of a useful life. He needed encouragement to find another purpose. He also worried about money.

Patients on home haemodialysis do not lead a normal life. Without a strong family for support and qualified caring staff to help, accidents and breakdowns happen. Teaching the hard facts of coping with haemodialysis for life is often mismanaged in renal units. The psychological needs of the patient and his family, and their need to understand future treatment and management, are much neglected subjects.

Michael died suddenly at home early in 1988. He was 56 years old.

Rowan Worsman, SEN, works in the Coronary Care Unit at the Royal Lancaster Infirmary

The power supply

RESOURCE 2

Patricia Lyne, Biochemistry, Session Five – The power supply, The Open Learning Foundation ,1994

1: The need for energy

Energy is a difficult thing to describe. We can't observe it directly; we can only observe its effects. Energy enables work to be performed.

In everyday life, we are involved in or affected by many different kinds of work, all of which require an input of energy. If you boil a kettle, drive a car or switch on a light, work is being performed. As you read this text, your body is engaged in many different kinds of work, even if you're sitting quite still. I would like to begin this session by considering some of the forms of work which cells undertake.

Varieties of work

In order to introduce cellular work, perhaps we could identify some everyday kinds of work and energy.

ACTIVITY 30

You can either think through this activity or actually carry it out.

Suppose that you have decided to take a break from work at this moment. You get up, go into the kitchen and make a cup of coffee. During this process, you will carry out several different kinds of activity or work and use household equipment to do other kinds. Make a short list of those that you can identify and the source of energy which makes that work possible.

Type of work   Source of energy

Commentary

You'll have made the coffee in your own particular way but, without doubt, some of the following kinds of work will have taken place.

- Mechanical work: getting up from the chair and moving around the house requires an input of muscular energy.

- Transport work: carrying objects such as cups and pans around also requires muscular energy. It is another form of mechanical work.

- Thermal work: boiling a kettle or heating a pan both require an input of heat energy, supplied either by electricity or by burning a fuel such as gas.

- Chemical work: as you stir or percolate the coffee, it undergoes a change.

The aroma becomes stronger and the solid material dissolves in the liquid. This also needs thermal energy.

- Electrical work: if you switch on the light, electrical energy is converted in the light bulb into the radiant energy of visible light.

All these kinds of work need an input of energy from some source. In each case, the source you have identified is not the original source of the energy. All forms of energy which we use to do everyday work represents a **conversion** of the original source into something which we can use.

For example, suppose that the electricity you use is produced in a hydroelectric power station. Where is the original source of the energy? One answer is in the mass of water confined behind a dam. As it is released, it causes turbines to rotate and generate electrical energy. We could not make direct use of the water in the dam to boil a kettle, but we can use it after its energy has been converted to another form.

Energy conversion

If you think about the power station example again, you may well conclude that the answer offered is only a partial one. It still leaves the question of how the water came to be behind the dam in the first place – and therefore how it came to have the energy which propels it through the turbines.

The more complete answer is that its energy came from the sun, which raised water vapour from the earth's surface into the clouds, from where it fell as rain in the hills. Its presence in the dam is the result of a series of **energy conversions**, starting in the sun.

Almost all the energy we use arises from the same source – **solar energy**, which enables plants to grow.

This is converted into the **chemical energy** which holds atoms together in the macromolecules made by plants. Over time, the plants die and decay to form fossil fuels – oil, coal and gas. The chemical energy from the plant material remains in the chemical structure of these fuels. When coal is used in a power station, its chemical energy is converted into electrical energy which, in its turn, can then be converted into other types such as mechanical energy or light.

The human diet contains material from both plant and animal sources. Animals rely on plants, either directly or indirectly, for their food. So the solar energy which forms the chemical bonds in plant materials is the source of all the chemical energy in our food.

These relationships are shown in *Figure 12*.

You may notice that all the kinds of energy shown in this diagram can be traced back to the sun – to solar energy. At various stages in the pathways, one kind of energy is changed to another. Such a step is termed energy conversion. These steps are of the utmost importance because they allow a natural source of energy – the sun – to be used to sustain life.

Human inventiveness has produced many **energy conversion systems**. We can convert the chemical energy of petrol into mechanical energy via a car engine and

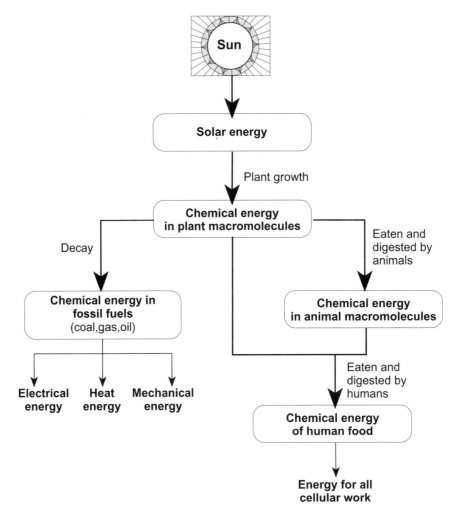

Figure 12 The relationship between sources of energy

electrical energy into light by means of an electric light bulb. Many of the pieces of equipment that we use at home or at work are energy converters. They change one form of energy into another which is useful for a particular purpose. Without an energy converter the chemical energy in petrol couldn't help us move from place to place, nor would the electrical energy passing through a wire help us to see in the dark.

When an energy converter operates, it is never 100 per cent efficient. Only a proportion of the energy that goes in as one form emerges as the useful output form. The rest is wasted, usually as heat – which can be thought of as 'useless' energy, unless it is being deliberately produced by the system. In a car engine, for example, the heat must be removed by the cooling system – but some of it is useful as a means of heating the interior of the car on cold days.

Living cells also have to convert energy. Their primary source is the chemical energy in food materials which, as shown in *Figure 12*, originates in solar energy. Living cells have to convert this chemical energy into a useful form and to deal with the waste heat produced.

The **mitochondria** are the structures in which this energy conversion takes place, and we will describe them in detail later. But before that, I would like to review the kinds of work for which the cell needs this useful energy, since this will increase your understanding of the problems which the living energy converters must solve.

Work in the cell

In *Activity 30*, you identified several kinds of work that are familiar in everyday life. Now let's see if there are parallels inside the living cell.

ACTIVITY 31

Looking back at *Activity 30*, list the kinds of work which were identified there. Next, using the knowledge you have so far acquired in this unit, decide if cells carry out a similar type of work. You might like to record your answers in *Table 4*.

In some cases, you may already be able to state how cells carry out a particular type of work. If so, include this in the table. If not, put a question mark in pencil next to the item.

Type of work	In what way, if any, do cells do this type of work?
Mechanical	
Transport	
Thermal	
Chemical	
Electrical	

Table 4 Work done in the cell

Commentary

At this stage in the unit, you should have realised that muscle cells move by contracting, so they do mechanical work. Transport is carried out by red blood cells, which use haemoglobin to carry oxygen around the body.

All cells do chemical work, as they use enzymes to bring about chemical change. Thermal and electrical work may have been a bit more problematic, but you should be able to complete these items later on.

ACTIVITY 32

Are there any other forms of cellular work which we could add? Look back through the unit to see if you can identify any other kinds of cellular work that have been mentioned, and add them to *Table 4*.

Commentary

In Session Two we concentrated on what the ribosomes do within the cell. Their work is to manufacture proteins, so you could add building up proteins to your list in *Table 4*. We also mentioned building messenger RNA, and in Session Four we talked about building carbohydrates and fats. The general term used in biochemistry for building up large molecules from their component parts is synthesis. This is a type of chemical work.

We have described one way that substances get across cell boundaries, in Session Four, as active transport. This too requires energy and is a form of work, so it should be another addition to your table, in the transport section.

Summary

- Energy enables work to be performed.

- There are many different forms of work and energy.

- Almost all the energy we use in our daily lives has its origin in solar energy.

- Energy may be changed from one form to another through an energy conversion system.

- The object of energy conversion is to produce a form of energy which can be used for a specific purpose.

- Living cells must carry out energy conversions. Their energy comes, ultimately, from the sun.

- Cells carry out energy conversions to produce forms of energy which can be used to do cellular work.

We are starting to build up a picture of the living cell as a small business, carrying out many kinds of work. It needs energy supplies for all of them. The remarkable thing is that living cells use a single energy source for all these diverse activities – just one energy source powers all these kinds of work. Let's look at this next.

The cell's energy source

Under the conditions existing in the human body – that is, under normal physiological conditions – our cells can carry out many different kinds of work. You've already listed some of these in *Table 4*.

All these sorts of work need energy. The single form of energy used by our cells is a substance called **adenosine triphosphate (ATP)** which is uniquely able to provide the energy for a wide range of cellular activities and to be regenerated after use within the cell itself. It is a truly wonderful and effective source of energy.

ATP allows things to happen which would normally be physiologically impossible. For example, to start to make a protein artificially, we would need to join together two amino acid molecules in the laboratory. This requires heat and the presence of other chemicals, and takes a long time. But enzymes on the ribosomes can join amino acids together very quickly at body temperature, as long as they have some ATP. In the cell, the ATP supplies the energy, whereas in the laboratory, the biochemist needs to heat the reaction mixture.

ATP is a small molecule which consists of four parts. We don't need to consider the details of its structure; we can simply visualise it as having –

- a main section: the **adenosine** (A) portion

with

- three smaller sections: the **phosphate** (P) portions

– linked to the main section. Take a look at *Figure 13*.

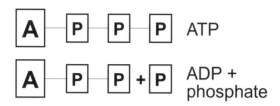

Figure 13 A model representing ATP

When ATP is used to provide energy for cellular work – to join amino acids together during protein synthesis, for example – it loses the last phosphate in the chain of three and becomes **adenosine diphosphate**, or **ADP** for short, as in the second part of *Figure 13*. ADP cannot be used as an energy source, but it can be built up again into ATP when the conditions are right.

When the third phosphate of ATP is released, a large 'bundle' of energy is set free. This bundle can be picked up by the working parts of the cell, and used in all the kinds of work we have considered so far. The ATP energy is channelled into cellular work.

ACTIVITY 33

The purpose of this activity is to help you construct a mental picture of how ATP functions. It isn't easy to find a familiar analogy for this process, but I hope the following will help.

Think of an occasion when you have been involved in a piece of work with another person who needed to be encouraged or motivated. It may have been a child, a colleague, or a patient or client who needed a lot of input from you to carry out their task. Reflect for a moment on how it felt and then, in a couple of sentences, jot down your observations of the event.

Commentary

Several people who tried this activity said that they felt 'drained' after putting a lot of effort into working with a person whose motivation for a particular task which had to be done was low. They felt that they were supplying all the energy needed both for themselves and the other person. Afterwards, they needed to be 'recharged' before they could give out again. Sometimes in health care, people give out so much in terms of physical and emotional energy that they suffer 'burn out', and need a long period of recharging.

The idea of 'giving out' to make things happen is one which we can apply to the way that ATP functions. This unique molecule has a structure which allows it to give out energy in just the right way to bring about work in the cell. In so doing, it becomes 'burnt out' (converted to ADP) and needs to be recharged before it can give out again.

I would like to try one more analogy to make the point clear. Imagine a see-saw with a person standing on one end. If someone else climbs to the top of a high wall nearby and jumps onto the other end of the see-saw, what will happen?

The first person will fly up into the air. Circus acrobats make use of this effect in some of their acts. Their jumps are controlled, just sufficiently to send the person on the other end of the see-saw flying off to the right height and distance. When the acrobat jumps, just the right amount of energy is released to produce the desired effect. ATP molecules do exactly this, so that cellular work is done in a controlled way.

ATP is used in all kinds of work, as I have already emphasised. But it is also produced from all the raw materials which enter the cell – the chemical energy from food is converted to ATP. So the cell is a lot more efficient than the small business, because it can satisfy all its energy needs by the production and use of this single source, instead of dealing with many different ones such as electricity, gas, petrol and so on, which involve numerous energy conversions.

Summary

- Living cells perform many different kinds of work.

- ATP is the energy source for all of them. It is produced from all kinds of food.

- After providing energy for cellular work, ATP is converted to 'useless' ADP and must be recharged before it can be used again.

Now that you have some information about the nature of the cell's energy source and the way that it is used, we need to consider how it is formed in more detail. To do this, we must go back to just inside the 'factory gates' and see what happens to the raw materials which are brought in to the cell, as it is their chemical energy which is destined to become ATP energy.

2: The fuel supply

Using glucose

In the previous session, we looked at how food macromolecules are broken down into their basic components. These components are then available for use by the cell, and they may:

- be synthesised into cellular products

- stored

or

- used as fuel for the mitochondrial power stations.

Here, I would like to consider the third of these options – what happens when the food components are used as fuel.

Glucose is the main supply of fuel for the cell. As you have already seen, it is produced when carbohydrate macromolecules are broken down during digestion.

When carbohydrates are digested to glucose, some of the energy holding their components together is set free as heat, which is used to maintain body temperature. It is used to perform thermal work. However, most of the original energy which formed the macromolecule remains locked up in the bonds holding together the atoms in the glucose molecules. When glucose enters the cell, it undergoes a process of rearrangement which enables that energy to be passed on to form ATP. Let's look in more detail at what happens to glucose during this process.

Splitting glucose

First of all, a series of enzymes working in sequence act on the glucose.

These enzymes change each glucose molecule into two molecules of **pyruvic acid**. Each glucose molecule has six carbon atoms and each pyruvic acid molecule has three.

We have summed this up in a single sentence, but it is actually a very complex series involving ten separate steps, each one carried out by a specialised enzyme. The sequence is called **glycolysis**, which literally means 'sugar splitting' because the six-carbon sugar molecule is split into two three-carbon molecules. The energy released in this splitting process is used to make two molecules of ATP for each molecule of glucose. In addition, each glucose molecule loses four atoms of hydrogen.

Equation 1

$$C_6H_{12}O_6 + 2ADP + 2P \quad\rightarrow\quad 2 \times C_3H_4O_3 + 2ATP + 4H$$

(glucose)   (enzymes of (pyruvic acid)
        glycolysis)

You will see from this equation that oxygen doesn't play any part at this stage. Glycolysis does not need any oxygen. It allows the cell to produce a small quantity of ATP in the absence of oxygen. We'll have a practical demonstration of this in the next activity, but first let's summarise some of the key facts about glycolysis, and explain what this equation means.

Summary

- In order to make use of the energy in the glucose, its molecules must be rearranged so that the energy can be handed on to ATP.

- In the cell, the first stage in the use of glucose is a series of ten steps, each brought about by a specialised enzyme.

- The overall process is called glycolysis. It does not require the presence of oxygen.

- Glycolysis results in each glucose molecule being split into two three-carbon molecules (pyruvic acid) and releasing four atoms of hydrogen.

- Glycolysis results in the production of a small amount of ATP. (Two molecules of ATP are gained for each molecule of glucose used).

Using equations

Equations such as *Equation 1* are used to convey information about chemical and biochemical change. The essential feature of an equation is that it balances. In other words, there must be the same number of atoms on each side of the arrow.

This equation tells us that each molecule of glucose splits into two molecules of pyruvic acid. A molecule of the latter has three atoms of carbon, four of hydrogen and three of oxygen. So two molecules of pyruvic acid account for six carbon, eight hydrogen and six oxygen atoms. Four hydrogen atoms are left over from the glucose molecule, which we write as 4H – indicating that these atoms have been liberated from the glucose in some way.

The equation also tells us that, during the splitting process, two molecules of ADP have been recharged to form ATP. Some of the energy holding the sugar molecule together has been used to form ATP from ADP and phosphate.

Please remember that *Equation 1* is a summary of ten separate steps in which the molecules of glucose are rearranged in order to allow this to happen. All ten steps are necessary if this part of the sugar's energy content is to be used efficiently and not wasted.

Working without oxygen

Glycolysis doesn't need any oxygen. It produces a small amount of ATP for each glucose molecule, and it produces free hydrogen atoms.

In the absence of oxygen, cells can produce a supply of ATP through glycolysis, which enables them to carry on working, as the next activity demonstrates.

ACTIVITY 34

This activity shows you what happens when cells work without oxygen. This really is a physical activity, so please only try it if you are fully fit.

First, raise one arm straight up in the air above your head, and let the other hand rest by your side. Clench both fists tightly, and then open out your fingers wide. Repeat this at the rate of once or twice a second. Try to keep clenching both fists at the same rate. Keep going for about five minutes, and record what you observe.

Stop and rest for a minute. Then try again, with the opposite arm raised this time. Again, record your observations.

Commentary

You probably noticed that the arm raised in the air became tired first, and that it was difficult to keep up the same rate of activity. Some people find that their dominant hand – the one they write with – is stronger than the other one in this exercise but that, even so, it is much harder to keep going with this hand when it is raised than when it is dependent.

Why should this be so? We could say that the muscles are getting tired, but why should they get tired more quickly when the arm is raised?

The answer is that, by clenching and unclenching the fist rapidly, we are making muscles work hard and using up the available ATP which is supplying the energy for that work. As long as the blood is bringing oxygen to these muscles, they can work at this rapid rate. But if the blood cannot bring so much oxygen, once the existing supply is used up we are making the muscles work in the absence of oxygen – in other words, **anaerobically**. Under these circumstances, glycolysis can take place producing a small energy output.

This allows the muscles to keep going if the exercise is not too violent, but it incurs a penalty. Do you remember those four hydrogen atoms in the glycolysis equation? During glycolysis, more and more hydrogen atoms accumulate. They clog up the system and, unless they are removed, it will seize up completely. Before this happens, as a last resort, the free hydrogen atoms can be transferred to pyruvic acid itself. Each molecule can accept two hydrogen atoms to produce lactic acid, as shown in *Equation 2*.

Equation 2

$$C_3H_4O_3 + 2H \qquad \longrightarrow \qquad C_3H_6O_3$$

(pyruvic acid)　　　(lactate dehydrogenase)　　　(lactic acid)

This allows the muscle to continue to work for longer still but, in time, the lactic acid itself will accumulate. It is a by-product of glycolysis, and alters the environment in which the enzymes of glycolysis work. When its level in muscle fibres begins to rise, these enzymes slow down until finally glycolysis stops, no more ATP can be produced and the muscle cannot contract any more. If you continued *Activity 34* for a longer period, you would find that it eventually became totally impossible to clench your raised hand because the muscle could no longer contract.

Lactic acid can easily pass out of muscle cells and into the bloodstream, so it is removed from exercising muscle where the blood supply is good. However, it begins to build up in the plasma, lowering its pH and producing **acidosis**. This can arise from several causes other than exercise. For example, if the blood supply to a tissue is poor, lactic acid can accumulate. Or in diabetes, excessive use of fat as an energy source produces ketones, which are also acidic and easily diffuse into the bloodstream.

If the plasma becomes more acidic in this way, it liberates carbon dioxide (CO_2) from one of the minerals in the plasma – bicarbonate. The result is that the blood then carries an extra load of carbon dioxide gas. This is detected by the nervous system and the rate of breathing is increased to enable the carbon dioxide to be blown off from the lungs.

When a person exercises vigorously, their breathing rate increases for these reasons. You may have noticed that when you have been exercising you continue to breathe hard after you have stopped. This is because the lactic acid is still present in your blood until it has been disposed of in the liver and you need to continue to get rid of carbon dioxide.

It is important for nurses to understand what is happening in the muscles and bloodstream when caring for a person with respiratory problems. When the oxygen supply in the blood is limited by conditions such as chronic bronchitis, emphysema and cystic fibrosis – all conditions which reduce the amount of oxygen the blood can carry – then there will be a shortage of oxygen in the muscles, and sustained muscular effort will be impossible.

Summary

- Glycolysis can occur anaerobically – that is, in the absence of oxygen.

- Cells can carry on working without oxygen, using the small amount of ATP produced in glycolysis.

- However, if the cells have to work hard, the hydrogen atoms produced in glycolysis build up.

- They can be mopped up by pyruvic acid, but this is only a temporary remedy, as this will produce lactic acid which slows down enzyme activity if it accumulates.

- Lactic acid passes out into the bloodstream. This causes acidosis and an increase in the rate of breathing.

- People with respiratory problems may have difficulty getting enough oxygen to their cells, so may have to rely on anaerobic ATP production. Sustained activity is very difficult under these conditions.

Into the 'power station'

We have described what happens to glucose in the absence of oxygen. Most of the time there is plenty of oxygen, delivered regularly to our tissues in the blood. Under these circumstances, the pyruvic acid and the hydrogen produced in glycolysis enter the mitochondria, where most of the chemical energy from the original glucose molecules is used to make a lot more ATP. It is important to emphasise that these two products of glycolysis, pyruvic acid and hydrogen, still retain most of that original energy.

The mitochondria are often called the 'power stations' of the cell. They are its main energy converters, because they take in pyruvic acid and hydrogen, which carry chemical energy from glucose, and produce ATP, which is the energy source that the cell can use.

When oxygen is plentiful in the cell, the 'gates' of the power stations open to admit the products of glycolysis.

Next, we will take a detailed look at the mitochondria to see what happens there.

The Clinical Nurse Specialist in intensive care

RESOURCE 3A

*Brenda Atkinson,
Nursing,
December 21, 1989-
January 10, 1990,
vol 4; no 1*

Though it has been slow to develop, there is now a distinct role for the specialist nurse in intensive care, says Belinda Atkinson.

'Developed appropriately the role of the CNS could . . . emerge as one of paramount importance'

During the past decade the role of the clinical nurse specialist (CNS) has been debated frequently in the literature from various aspects.

The original concept was developed in the United States more than 20 years ago. Development of the role in the UK has been slow, and not aided by various NHS reorganisations. These enhanced the administrative role of senior nursing staff at the expense of the clinical one[1].

However, this is not true of all branches of nursing and some specialities have been instrumental in developing a specialist role; for example, there are well established stoma care nurses, infection control nurses and breast care counsellors.

Thompson and Webster[2] attempt to distinguish between nurse specialists and clinical nurse specialists: 'A nurse specialist is a nurse who has chosen to specialise in a certain aspect of nursing and a clinical nurse specialist would appear to be a nurse specialist who has chosen to do this within the clinical setting.' A considerable degree of overlap is to be expected. Consequently, the role of the clinical nurse specialist needs careful clarification.

Balcombe[3] says the CNS should develop patient services for a specific client group; be a clinically based leader for the nursing team; develop nursing expertise within the unit; provide advice on nursing care and developments; and offer therapeutic counselling for patients and staff. Barrie-Shevlin[4] suggests the four major components of the role are clinical practice, education, consultation and research.

The RCN[5] defines the nurse specialist as: 'someone who demonstrates refined clinical practice as a result of significant experience, advanced expertise, or knowledge of a particular nursing branch or speciality'. It further suggests that, to claim true status as a specialist, the nurse must be involved in clinical practice, consultation, teaching, management and research.

Thompson and Webster[2] suggest that nurses working in critical care areas often tend to think of themselves, and are thought of by others, as specialists in their chosen field. The Oxford English Dictionary defines a specialist as 'one who devotes himself to a particular branch of a profession'. Thompson and Webster say it is true that critical care nurses concentrate on certain unique aspects of patient treatment and care, though the viewpoint from which they do this may be debatable.

What scope is there, therefore, for the CNS in the intensive care unit (ICU)? Barrie-Shevlin's suggested components of the role provide a framework upon which to examine this further[4].

The CNS should be instrumental in the maintenance of high standards of care and practice in the ICU. In addition to education, there are two major ways in which she may achieve this. First, she is involved in the process of nursing; the assessment, planning, delivery and evaluation of the care given to patients and their families.

Role model

Markham[6] proposes that, in this respect, the CNS acts as a role model for other nurses, demonstrating knowledge, skill and abilities at an advanced level.

The role model effect is often underestimated. This is because unless teaching sessions, for example, are formal and obviously organised, staff may not feel they are receiving (or 'doing') training.

In effect, they are. All experienced staff must be aware they will become a role model in the ICU environment. Generally, the higher up the ladder one goes, the more one is watched, copied and learned from in this way.

In addition, the CNS needs to become involved in the setting of standards, policies and procedures relating both to the direct care setting in ICU and to more general hospital standards and policies which may have an effect on the ICU. Ideally, the CNS should be a resource person to the unit in which she is based and also available to advise on the care of critically ill patients elsewhere in the hospital.

Setting standards for use in the clinical area both helps to evaluate the care provided for patients, and supplies benchmarks for use in quality assurance programmes. Such programmes are becoming a fundamental part of health care today.

They need to be devised and implemented in conjunction with those involved in the actual hands-on delivery of care. The CNS seems ideally placed to facilitate this.

The market is awash with equipment and accessories for use in the care of critically ill patients. But how do we evaluate them? The CNS is in a perfect position to match product to patient; to arrange trials of products in the clinical field; to evaluate and advise managers accordingly.

The CNS, then, must set and demonstrate high standards of clinical practice; advise on the setting of policy and procedure; keep abreast of current advances in technology and practice; and strive to constantly improve ways of delivering patient care.

Barrie-Shevlin[4] suggests that, as a teacher and facilitator of knowledge, the CNS must be able to answer 'how and why' questions and recognise opportunities for on the spot teaching: 'She must be prepared to assist with both nurses' and patient's problems and keep abreast of change and current research into nursing practice.'

Today, education is complex. It has been suggested that education is responding to the pressures of society, and undergoing change in the same way as nursing. Nurse education does not stop at the end of basic training. Snow[8] wrote that: 'All critical care nurses have a need for educational offerings.'

Boyes[9] states: 'Those involved in education are challenged in educating the nurse of the future; to prepare nurses for creativity and flexibility; to teach the nurse not everything there is to learn, but to teach the nurse how to learn – to be prepared to face change and to develop in a flexible way when change occurs.' This philosophy was first advanced by Florence Nightingale[10] who wrote: 'I do not pretend to teach her – I ask her to teach herself, and for this purpose I venture to give her some hints.'

Education

The scope for the CNS in the realm of education is immense. Her function as a role model in direct clinical practice has already been discussed. In the clinical area this can be extended into formal group teaching sessions; one-to-one bedside teaching sessions; involvement in the orientation of new staff to the workplace; development of a mentor system; assessment of basic and post-basic nurses in training; and arrangement of educational programmes for visitors to the unit.

Assessing skills

In addition, she may encourage members of staff to pursue courses in teaching and assessing skills, such as the increasingly popular ENB 998 course, 'Teaching and assessing in clinical practice', or the City and Guilds 730 course, the Further Education Teachers' Certificate.

Intensive care is developing rapidly as a speciality, as technology expands therapeutic possibilities. There is, therefore, a great need for on-going educational programmes and a competent individual who is able to assist staff to relate their theoretical knowledge to the realities of clinical practice. With the advent of changes in nurse education, it is likely this need will increase.

The CNS has a role in liaison with other specialities and disciplines. This can be seen as twofold. She has a consultative role to critically ill patients in other areas of the hospital. This could involve either advising directly on patient care or acting as a resource person in identifying other appropriate agencies. In the 'outgoing' aspects of the role there is also a place for the promotion of the speciality of intensive care nursing on a more general basis – acting both in career guidance and in recruitment aspects.

The role is also twofold in the ICU. She must be available for consultation by nursing staff and by staff of other disciplines. To this effect, she must be perceived as credible on the grounds of her knowledge base and clinical skills. This will mean that, as part of her role, she should be devoting time to nursing[2]. She must also act as a co-ordinator for outside agencies and know what support services are available and how to use them appropriately.

Research

Research is a fundamental part of the role if we are to advance the practice of intensive care nursing on a scientific basis. The systematic enquiry on which research is based is vital if all other aspects of the work are to be successfully developed[4]. The CNS should be actively involved in research and promote awareness of the importance of research for nursing practice.

A positive attitude towards research engendered early in the intensive care nurse's experience helps increase motivation to become actively involved in future studies. In addition, post-basic clinical courses contain an appreciation of the research component in the curriculum. Diploma and degree courses are now more widely accessible. The CNS could act as a valuable facilitator and resource for staff undertaking such courses.

The literature agrees on the desirable

qualifications and personal qualities of a CNS. Markham[6] advocates a combination of national board clinical courses, FETC and the 'Understanding and appreciation of research' course. Though she believes this is no substitute for preparation at degree level, she sees it as a basis for growth and development.

Thompson and Webster[2] agree that possession of post-basic qualifications are desirable and further recommend possession of the Diploma in Nursing. Balcombe[11] agrees with this suggestion. It therefore seems the ideal preparation includes a degree in nursing or diploma in nursing (revised curriculum); a relevant national board course in the appropriate clinical speciality; and a teaching qualification.

Personal attributes

As to personal qualities, Thompson and Webster[2] describe the CNS as needing to be 'imaginative, creative, and innovative, as well as strong-willed and purposeful'. Balcombe[3,11] mentions the need for problem-solving, communication, counselling and caring skills, plus an ability to recognise and cope with stress.

Markham[6] discusses leadership abilities and communication skills, and Walker[12] says the CNS must have administrative support to function successfully as a consultant. Finally, Barrie-Shevlin[4] considers essential personal skills to be creativity, enthusiasm, charm and diplomacy.

The concept of the CNS in the UK was proposed by the RCN[13] following the Briggs report. There is no doubt the idea has become a reality in certain areas – notably those where the CNS has been allowed flexibility to work and not necessarily tied to the bureaucratic structure of the health service and the confines of the hospital setting. Examples include nurses working with diabetics, in breast care, stoma care and nutrition.

There are two main complications in the ICU. The multidisciplinary nature of the work, and the high priority placed on such teamwork, make it difficult to claim exclusive specialist areas. And, until now, many attempts at creating such posts in the ICU have been combined with an administrative function. This makes the division of time difficult, often with the need for a substantially greater bias towards the administrative aspects of the role.

Despite the current pressures and uncertainty surrounding the health service, these are exciting and challenging times for nursing. The next decade will see radical changes in administrative and educational aspects of nursing. Developed appropriately, the role of the CNS could, as a result, emerge as one of paramount importance.

Many current hospital administrative structures have led to a broadening of the role of those previously in charge of clinical areas to take on more administrative aspects such as financial management. This has led to the need for a professional advisory structure, both at hospital and individual clinical area level. This development has largely been recognised by the clinical grading structure, with particular emphasis on the G, H and I grades. It has thus enabled the retention of senior nursing expertise in the clinical areas.

Changes in the delivery of care, such as the implementation of primary nursing, may lead to a radical change in role for senior nurses – from supervisor to resource and advisory person. An experienced individual is needed, therefore, to facilitate this shift in role and advise and support primary nurses in the delivery of care.

Project 2000

Project 2000 calls for similar expertise, to facilitate changes in skill mix and learning patterns appropriate to the clinical area. Balcombe[3,11] describes the need to establish a learning resource centre, where staff can find facilities for study and information. The CNS has a role in the provision of such a resource centre, the education of learners and the support of staff in their role as mentors and facilitators.

Finally, the CNS has a role in the audit of care and quality assurance exercise. She will set the bench marks to facilitate measurement and, being clinically based, is well placed to monitor attainment and maintenance of standards of care. Recent reports, such as that of the King's Fund Panel[14], have highlighted the deficit in audit of intensive care. The CNS could have a valuable role in remedying this lack of information.

Developed appropriately, the future for the CNS in intensive care could at last look encouraging. Nursing has seen great changes recently and it seems likely that its demands and complexities will further increase. The CNS must be able to manipulate the diverse elements of her role, working within the difficult and complex environment of the ICU to provide the best possible care for critically ill patients and their families.

Belinda Atkinson, RGN, RSCN, DipN (Lond). is Clinical Services Manager, Intensive Care Units, Southampton General Hospital.

References

1. Salmon, B (1966) Report of the Committee on Senior Nursing Staff Structure (Salmon report), HMSO.

2. Thompson, D R & Webster, R A (1986) 'The clinical nurse specialist in critical care', *Nursing Practice*, 1, 236-241.

3. Balcombe, K (1989) 'Prime time for development', *Nursing Standard*, January, 3;17, 36-37.

4. Barrie-Shevlin, P (1985) 'Creativity, enthusiasm, diplomacy', *Nursing Mirror*, May, 160;20, 46-47.

5. RCN (1988) Specialities in Nursing, RCN.

6. Markham, G (1988) 'Special cases', *Nursing Times*, June, 84;26, 29-30.

7. Jarvis, P (1986) A Sociology of Lifelong Education and Lifelong Learning, Department of Adult Education, University of Georgia.

8. Snow, J L (1983) 'Care of the critically ill child – is there a better way?', in Stahler-Miller, K, Neonatal and Paediatric Critical Care Nursing, New York, Churchill Livingstone.

9. Boyes, M (1987) 'Intensive care nursing education', *Nursing*, 3;16, 593-596.

10. Nightingale, F (1924) Notes on Nursing, Harrison & Sons.

11. Balcombe, K (1989) 'Leading the way', *Nursing Standard*, January, 3;16, 21.

12. Walker, M L (1986) 'The clinical nurse specialist as a consultant', *Nursing Management*, 7;5, 61.

13. RCN (1975) New Horizons in Clinical Nursing, RCN.

14. King's Fund (1989) Intensive Care in the UK: Report from the King's Fund Panel, May, King's Fund Institute.

Further reading

Shuldham, C (1986) 'The nurse on the intensive care unit', *Intensive Care Nursing*, 1;4, 181-186.

RESOURCE 3B

Joanne Whelton, Nursing, December 21, 1989-January 10, 1990, vol 4; no 1

The midwife and foetal medicine

The development of diagnostic medicine in antenatal care has led to a specialised role for some midwives, says Joanne Whelton.

'It is necessary to…help families decide whether prenatal screening is a viable proposition'.

The growth of prenatal screening and management within obstetrics has created a role for the midwife within this new area.

Just as the midwife providing routine antenatal care offers advice and support for screening such as serum alphafetoprotein, and more recently HIV testing, the midwife involved with prenatal diagnosis on a full-time basis is able to provide midwifery care with advice and support for mothers requiring tests undertaken within the foetal medicine unit. Her role complements that of the medical staff and is similar to that of the midwife working in the antenatal clinic.

But what of the skills developed by the midwife within the field of prenatal diagnosis? Does her experience warrant her owning the title of 'clinical nurse/midwife specialist'?

Technological developments in obstetrics have radically changed the medical management of pregnancy. Today the use of ultrasound as a screening method is offered routinely to most pregnant women. However, as midwives, do we ever really stop to question the implications of such a procedure?

Should we favour ultrasound scans without further thought or should we all take time to consider our own perceptions and thoughts on prenatal diagnosis before we advise mothers? I sincerely believe that we must all take the responsibility for the development of our own understanding and feelings. Such awareness is crucial for the midwife specialist within foetal medicine.

Prenatal diagnosis is a screening facility for any pregnant mother at risk of delivering a baby with an abnormality. Foetal medicine is the management offered upon detection of problems which, with therapy, may result in a successful outcome; for example, rhesus isoimmunisation and foetal urinary obstruction.

Inevitably, most midwives are involved in some form of prenatal screening. In the antenatal clinic, discussion regarding serum alphafetoprotein testing requires the same understanding of possible implications should any deviation from a normal result occur.

Fortunately, today we are more aware of the need for informed consent from the parents before undertaking such tests, and recognition of the parents' choice to opt out of screening should they wish to do so. But can we be sure parents are always provided with the information and unbiased support to facilitate their decision? Can we be sure pressures are not put on them to conform, or that other screening tests are not then arranged as an alternative, such as a scan to exclude a neural tube defect?

Professor Stuart Campbell of King's College Hospital was among the first to acknowledge the potential of ultrasound scanning in the screening of pregnant mothers, and has always described ultrasound as providing us with a 'window to the womb', enabling us to monitor the well-being of the foetus.

Is the ultrasound department an area in which the midwife has an important place or is this too great an extension of her role?

I believe the midwife can make a valuable contribution within this area. A few centres already have midwives based in their scan departments – in some instances co-ordinating the service of it.

In an attempt to help develop the skills of the midwife in carrying out basic measurement scans, training courses are offered in one of the leading London hospitals. The interest shown by midwives is great but the tradition of radiographers alone, rather than united with the obstetricians and midwives together managing the service in the ultrasound department, has made it difficult for midwives to penetrate this area.

Surely the midwife's obstetric and basic knowledge of maternal and foetal anatomy enables her, with adequate training and experience, to become fully competent to an acceptable level to work as a member of the ultrasound department team? The communication skills the midwife develops during her work are also of benefit to such a department.

We can all probably recall occasions when mothers have waited in the ultrasound department when a problem was found while the doctor was 'tied up' and the radiographer was not in a position to discuss details with the woman. Such situations result in an anxious period for all concerned.

When a facility is provided within a unit for detection of possible anomalies – after all, is that not why scans are undertaken? – surely the least we can aim to provide is adequate support and help when such a problem arises, by providing midwives with counselling experience to be there. The midwife, in her capacity of ensuring the best possible care for the mother, is able to offer support during the discussion with medical staff and then throughout any decision-making period which may follow.

The use of ultrasound provided not only a window but also opened the door as far as foetal medicine was concerned. It

has enabled such tests an amniocentesis, cordiocentesis (foetal blood sampling from the umbilical cord) and chorionic villus sampling. Today, amniocentesis is provided for mothers nationally, and chorionic villus sampling is developing rapidly as an alternative to amniocentesis. Cordiocentesis, meanwhile, remains restricted to specialist centres.

For six years, I worked as a midwife alongside pioneers in this field – doctors attempting to develop techniques of management for conditions which threatened the survival of the yet unborn child. I extended my role as a midwife to include the ability to carry out basic ultrasound screening, to care for mothers during the operative procedure itself, and to develop the necessary counselling and support skills to enable them to cope with the ordeal of facing such screening. Thus was created a clinical nurse specialist within the new area of foetal medicine.

It has really been in the past 25 years that prenatal ultrasound screening has been offered, but only in the past 10-15 years has it become more readily available throughout the country. The initial equipment was expensive and large, but with technological advances the manufacturers were able to produce smaller, more mobile machines capable of producing imagery of outstanding quality. This enabled the experienced eye to visualise the structural make-up of the foetus, allowing close scrutiny for anatomical defects.

The initial invasive diagnostic procedure was that of amniocentesis. The breakthrough in the understanding of the chromosomal structure and genetic make-up of the human being provided the knowledge required.

Placentesis was then attempted as a method of obtaining foetal blood for these studies. However, maternal contamination was frequent.

This was followed by foetoscopic foetal blood sampling which enabled a pure foetal blood sample to be aspirated. The use of a telescope introduced transabdominally allowed sampling of foetal blood from the umbilical cord, foetal skin and foetal liver. Foetal examination by direct visualisation was also possible.

The foetoscope was discarded as ultrasound equipment developed to the extent that the site for sampling was clearly recognisable by scan alone; hence, the procedure of cordiocentesis. Chorionic villus biopsy is the most recent development, providing a method of detecting genetically inherent disorders from eight weeks' gestation.

The vast proportion of antenatal mothers are now offered the opportunity to have an ultrasound examination of their foetus. But, rather than being 'offered a scan', would it be more accurate to say that their obstetricians request one, or that a scan is arranged for them?

Most mothers expect a scan and even look forward to the excitement of seeing their baby for the first time. How many consider that the scan is actually to exclude anomalies? What happens when an abnormality is revealed? The initial shock of facing the reality of abnormality can be devastating. Then, the midwife in the foetal medicine unit is the vital link.

A comprehension of genetics is useful for the midwife in the foetal medicine unit. Studies of foetal tissue to exclude autosomal recessive conditions and chromosomal defects form the basis of most work undertaken there. The appropriate liaison with specific departments enables the diagnoses of inherited disorders by determining the family carrier status. For several conditions family studies are crucial in interpreting the result of foetal screening.

Table 1 Conditions frequently encountered for prenatal diagnosis	
Haemaglobinopathies	- such as sickle cell anaemia and ß-thalassaemia
Coagulation disorders	- such as factor VIIIc deficiency (Haemophilia A) and factor IX deficiency (Haemophilia B)
Cystic fibrosis	
Duchenne muscular dystrophy	
Inborn errors of metabolism	- such as α 1anti-trypsin deficiency
Immunodeficiencies	- severe combined immuno-deficiency (SCID)
Rapid karyotype studies	- for example, for maternal age, following previous abnormality or for ultra-sound detected abnormality

Table 2 Procedures which may be used to diagnose or treat the foetus	
Foetal skin biopsy	- such as for epidermolysis bullosa letalis and albinism
Foetal liver biopsy	- such as for ornithine-carbamoyl-transferase deficiency
Management of rhesus iso-immunisation	
Management of obstruction of the renal tract	

Though the foetal medicine unit carries out the vital procedure of obtaining the sample from the foetus, the actual analysis of that tissue once acquired – for example, foetal blood, skin, liver or urine – is frequently carried out off-site in the appropriate department in specialist institutions.

Explanation to parents of the clinical significance of genetics, and its implications for the family, are frequently required. A knowledge of common and uncommon conditions has to be built up to enable understanding of the abnormality faced by the respective parents. It is also necessary to facilitate counselling and guidance as required to help families decide whether prenatal screening is a viable proposition for them.

The dilemma of whether to terminate a pregnancy presents both the midwife and parents with many questions. Both need to answer those to their own satisfaction before any decision can be made.

As we have seen, the midwife in the foetal medicine unit uses all her midwifery skills and more. Her role develops to that of a counsellor and an educator. Her prime concern is that of the safety and well-being of the mother and her unborn child as far as possible.

The skills she develops enable her to act as a liaison and co-ordinator. Her experience and knowledge should be shared not only with the mothers in her care, but also with colleagues and students. For instance, I have been asked to give lectures and lead discussions on prenatal diagnosis; ethical issues in foetal medicine; counselling and support of parents having babies with potential abnormalities; counselling skills for midwives; and the role of the midwife within foetal medicine. I have also been involved with the development of support groups for both parents and staff.

The final activity of the midwife specialist, once she has carried out her role of counsellor and co-ordinator of services, is to maintain statistical information of the work undertaken and to complete follow-up on mothers attending the unit. This follow-up of families is of great importance, especially in providing support should the outcome result in the loss of the baby whether as a consequence of confirmation of abnormality or, less commonly, from spontaneous abortion as direct consequence of the procedure. The risk association is usually quoted as less than three per cent for chorionic villus sampling, one to two per cent for cordiocentesis, and less than 0.5 per cent for amniocentesis.

Research is another important component. Whether medical or midwifery based, the midwife's role is to protect the mother and her baby at all times, but she must be able to innovate and develop the midwifery care she is able to provide in her capacity as a 'clinical midwife specialist' working as part of the foetal medicine team.

Joanne Whelton, SRN, SCM, Dip Counselling, is a senior midwife at University College Hospital, London.

The nature of dilemmas in dialysis nurse practice

RESOURCE 3C

*Sally Wellard,
Journal of Advanced
Nursing, 1992,
17, 951-959*

Dilemmas are a part of nurse practice. In situations where a problem potentially has two or more unsatisfactory resolutions, the nurse chooses which course of action to take. The decision to choose constitutes a dilemma. This study focuses on the dilemmas faced by nurses in dialysis units and the context in which they occur. A qualitative design was employed, using open interviews with eight nurses currently employed in dialysis nursing. This approach was taken in order to explore and gain in-depth understanding of the dilemmas in practice. Analysis reveals that dilemmas encountered in dialysis nursing emerge from conflicts in relationships with other people in the work environment. The dilemmas relate to the nurses' perception of the limited power they have in the determination of their practice. This powerlessness is reinforced by their perceived and real isolation from nurses working outside their area of practice. Traditionally, literature on dilemmas in nursing has focused on the development of ethical frameworks to guide practice and the resolution of dilemmas. However, the findings of this study suggest that if nurses are to deal with dilemmas effectively, both for the nurse and the patient, there must be an examination of the structural constraints affecting their practice. Models that are employed by nurses to guide practice must account for the structural elements in the work environment.

Introduction

Dilemmas in nursing have had considerable attention in nursing literature, but predominantly authors have written from the view of dilemma resolution for the 'ideal nurse'; that is, models for understanding and resolving dilemmas are derived from a theoretical stance. There has been little attempt to assess empirically the applicability of the models to the actual practice environment of nurses (Davis & Aroskar 1978, Felton & Parsons 1987, Thompson *et al.* 1983). This study sought to explore the nature of dilemmas encountered in dialysis nursing from the perspective of the nurse clinician/practitioner.

There has been a reliance on bioethical models applied to nursing to provide a foundation for the development of codes of practice, to guide practice and the resolution of ethical dilemmas. It has been assumed that the 'neon' issues of bioethics (for example, informed consent and refusal of treatment) are a feature of nurse practice (Evans 1986). However, there has been little critique of the relevance to practice of bioethics (Fry 1989).

Codes of practice, a recurring theme in nursing literature, posit that the nurse is autonomous and able to determine what actions are moral. Yet these codes, offered uncritically, assume the nurse has control over her/his work (Evans 1986). Muschamp (1989) argues that dilemmas for nurses emerge from situations where they experience themselves as being powerless.

The medical dominance of the health care sector reveals factors that may inhibit the nurse from acting as an autonomous moral agent. Willis (1989) describes three central components of medical dominance; autonomy, authority and sovereignty. The medical profession, he argues, has the power to control the practice of the members of its profession, and is able to maintain an effective monopoly over health care delivery. Its autonomy, in not being subject to 'direction and evaluation' (Willis 1989) by others, promotes an élite position in society for members of the medical profession. The authority of the medical profession over other health care workers is deterministic; doctors, legitimately empowered by the state, determine the direction of service, with other health workers in a subordinate role. The notion of the sovereignty of the medical profession is wide in its application. Society accepts the medical view of health as the legitimate model and places trust in doctors to determine the appropriate directions for health care (Willis 1989).

Medical power

Medical power over the delivery of health care structures the work environment of the nurse. Gender is an important dimension of control in the health care setting. The male-dominated medical profession maintains a superior, authoritarian role over the predominately female nursing profession, and this has promoted the use of the analogy of the family. The nurse as the mother figure, subservient to the doctor (husband), provides care to the sick and dependent patient (child). The role of the nurse is practical and manual, whereas the doctor is knowledgeable and scientific (Game & Pringle 1983, Turner 1987).

The nurse in this view is part of a group oppressed by the medical profession. Roberts (1983) suggests that oppression amongst nurses can be seen in the 'fact that nurses lack autonomy, accountability, and control over the nursing profession'. The major characteristics of oppressed groups include: perceiving the dominant group as more highly valued than themselves (in this case the nurse views medicine as more highly valued than nursing); a desire to become 'like' the dominant group that leads to low self-esteem and submissiveness; and inter-group conflict or 'horizontal violence' within the oppressed group as a result of being unable to revolt against the dominant group.

It is argued that nurses working in high dependency units experience environmental constraints which limit their choice of nursing actions. Nurses working in environments where technology is used to support and sustain life are referred to as high dependency nurses, that is, the patients in their care have a high dependency on the nurse and health care setting to 'survive' (McClelland 1985). Dialysis nursing is a high dependency area; patients are dependent on dialysis to survive and in turn dependent on the nurse to ensure their access to 'safe' dialysis.

Schaefer (1989) describes dilemmas in critical care as conflict between professional and personal values, between nurses and doctors, nurses and other health care workers and/or nurses and the institution. She states that 'often nurses have limited or no input into decisions that are made regarding the patients for whom they render care'. Rushton (1988) presents similar findings in neonatal intensive care.

There is limited discussion in nursing literature of the dilemmas encountered by dialysis nurses. Richmond (1986) describes the dialysis nurse as being 'usually involved in a chain of command that makes her the target for release of frustrations by physicians, supervisors and co-workers'. The uses of sophisticated technological treatments that are rapidly changing and caring for patients who have multiple system disease contribute to the complex work environment of these nurses.

The review of literature suggests that there has been little empirical investigation into the dilemmas experienced by dialysis nurses. It supports the need to consider the roles and relationships of nurses with medical staff, patients and co-workers in exploring the dilemmas experienced by dialysis nurses.

Methodology

Qualitative design used for this study allows in-depth understanding of the issues underlying dilemmas in practice. This design sought to explain the everyday issues of participants and the broader issues of structure and meanings (Angus 1986).

Some qualitative reports argue that the researcher should be objective or context free (Germain 1986). However, two major contextual elements brought to the study by the author are acknowledged. First, seven years of dialysis nursing experience before the study provided knowledge of the particular language and work patterns relating to the dialysis work environment. Therefore, the researcher had minimal difficulty with technical language and procedures, and participants were able to converse with minimal explanation. Second, a theoretical perspective that focuses on structure of the environment and its impact on nurse practice was applied.

Open interviews

Nurses currently practising in renal dialysis units were interviewed using an open interview technique. The snowball technique was employed to meet participants; that is, each of the participants suggested the next participant (Field & Morse 1985). Initial contact was by telephone and provided opportunity for a broad explanation of the study, the amount of time that participation would involve and the assurance of confidentiality if the nurse chose to participate. This strategy proved to be successful. Participants were asked not to discuss the content of the interview with their colleagues to avoid the creation of a group consensus before the interviews which were conducted in their own homes.

The three major themes that the interview sought to cover with participants were: their perceptions of the role of the dialysis nurse, the dilemmas encountered in dialysis nurse practice and coping strategies for dealing with such dilemmas. Questions that were incorporated into discussion were:

1. How long have you worked in dialysis, and why did you choose this area of nursing? What is good about dialysis nursing, what keeps you there?

2. What is your role in the unit? How is work organized? What do you do?

3. Are there problems you experience in trying to achieve your role? What issues

do nurses in your unit have to deal with?

4. How do you feel about these issues? What do you do to cope with these problems? Do some other nurses deal with these issues differently from you? Is that better?

This paper will discuss findings related to the dilemmas encountered in practice.

Ethical considerations for the researcher

The two major ethical issues considered were protection of participants and 'honest' analysis (Germain 1986, Parse *et al.* 1985). First, participants signed a consent form at the outset that clearly emphasized the voluntary nature of participation. Confidentiality was assured. The individual's identity has not been linked to the data, and pseudonyms have been employed in presentation of all data. Participants were also assured that their employing hospital would not be identified. This was of concern to most of the participants as the dialysis community in Victoria is very 'small' and linking individuals to the study would be relatively simple if the unit were identifiable. Second, the integrity of this study is reliant on the faithful representation of the data and avoidance of distortion by omission of data (Opie 1989).

Analysis

All data collected were considered and the research process sought to uncover themes or patterns from the content (German 1986). Analysis commenced during transcription and, with subsequent readings, themes were identified.

Selection of quotations from text that are more than just illustrative proved useful in analysis (Opie 1989). Four aspects of spoken text were considered: intensity of speech, contradictory moments, emotional tone and the use of whole sentences instead of recursive speech. After preliminary themes were identified, analysis focused on re-reading the transcripts to locate the themes and to note exceptions to the themes. The task of analysis then moved to interpretation. Discovery of meanings required interaction between the data and theory, to determine whether current theory could explain the findings or if new theoretical propositions were needed.

Seeking rigour

The scientific adequacy of analysis and the subsequent conclusions drawn are fundamental in seeking rigour. Qualitative research views truth as relative. Four criteria for assessing scientific adequacy are credibility, fittingness, auditability and confirmability (Sandelowski 1986). Each

of the criteria was met. Several participants were asked to read the preliminary findings, which they acknowledged as reflective of their experience. The presentation of a paper to a broad nursing audience not participating in this study provided an opportunity for confirming a 'fit' with the reality of their lived experience. Auditability has been facilitated through the careful storage of tapes, transcripts and notes from interviews and preliminary analysis.

Findings

Eight female nurses were interviewed, all currently employed in metropolitan renal units that provide dialysis to patients with chronic or acute renal failure. The time employed in dialysis ranged from nine months to eight years. Two were employed in senior positions, one as a charge nurse and the other as associate charge nurse, in different units. The education profiles of these nurses were similar. Only one participant had not completed a post-basic renal nursing course. Three of the nurses are currently undertaking further study; two in Bachelor of Applied Science (Nursing), the other in a management diploma for general business.

Nurse's role in dialysis

The nurses described their role in dialysis in terms of the tasks associated with monitoring dialysis treatment. All participants talked at length about the technical management of dialysis. They saw the role of the nurse as that of supervising dialysis treatments and teaching patients how to manage their own dialysis and symptoms related to complications of chronic renal failure and dialysis.

Dilemmas resulting from conflicts in relationships

The 'neon' issues of bioethics were not the major concerns in daily practice. Dilemmas were experienced by dialysis nurses, however, these dilemmas related to their perception of the power they have in determining the care they deliver. One nurse summarized this perception:

'Nurses don't have any control over it [dialysis], it's the people who devise the machines and the medical people, . . . we have a supportive role, just maintaining, keeping the system going.' (Barbara)

A consistent theme was that dilemmas occur for nurses where conflicts arise in relationships with others in the workplace. Five relationships were identified as conflicting and hence dilemmas occur. These are relationships between: patient and doctor, doctor and nurse, nurse and patient, nurse and nurse, nurse and administration. Dilemmas were seldom the exclusive domain of one particular relationship but implicated in many relationships.

In order to understand the nature of the conflicts and resultant dilemmas, each of the relationships, as perceived by the participants, is described.

Patient-doctor relationship

When nurses perceived a poor doctor-patient relationship, they experienced dilemmas. Primarily, these dilemmas involved having unclear means for resolving the inadequate relationship between these two parties. Nurses described experiencing dilemmas when they found that doctors had given poor and inadequate explanations to patients. Patients and families would seek clarification from the nurse, who frequently felt powerless to disclose information that was seen to be medical in nature.

Doctors reportedly gave scanty and sporadic follow-up to patients after treating the 'obvious' medical problems. Major acute problems were dealt with efficiently and effectively by the medical staff. However, the management of everyday mundane problems was seen as poor.

Nurses believed that they had little choice of action. They were concerned with betraying the trust they may have existed between the patient and their medical practitioner if they appeared to criticise the medical opinions and treatment options. Concern was also expressed about legal constraints regarding information the nurse may give about what they saw as medical matters.

Doctor-nurse relationship

All participants described conflict in their relationships with medical staff, which was the relationship discussed most frequently and in most depth. Dilemmas for the nurse emerged from seemingly unproductive and frequently conflicting relationships with medical staff.

Nurses described situations where access to expert medical knowledge was limited, creating many dilemmas. Nephrologists were seen by the dialysis nurse as having expert knowledge. Registrars and residents, however, were frequently seen as not having sufficient specific knowledge. In particular, these doctors were viewed as having little skill in the management of patients on dialysis. This frequently resulted in nurses undertaking responsibilities outside their job description.

Short medical rotations were described as producing low levels of knowledge and poor motivation amongst medical staff. As one nurse remarked:

'They have no idea what they are treating . . . he [the registrar] may wait for the physician to turn up, that might be next week. He [the registrar] might say use your discretion and do this; that really isn't good enough.' (Mary)

Consultant nephrologists, while open to discussing issues with the nursing staff, were generally not readily accessible. They communicated predominantly through the registrar, who decided the point at which the higher level of knowledge was needed. Registrars were frequently seen as excessively interventionist, and reluctant to seek advice from the consultants.

Nurses described situations where they perceived the medical staff as not accepting their nursing expertise as a valid and valuable contribution to treatment decisions. These situations included, first, the acceptance of new patients who proceed onto the chronic dialysis programme, second, the discussion of acute treatment options, and finally, the application of selection criteria for transplant candidates.

Some of the nurses identified their perspective as being different from the doctors' perspective. They saw their close relationships with patients as making them more subjective than medical staff. As one nurse said:

'Sometimes, if I talk too much, the doctor will think, who do you think you are, do you have the expertise? . . . most probably their point of view is different from mine because I am attached to the patient. For them there must be some other reasons.' (Milly)

Dilemmas also arose for nurses when they were expected to do work for which they had no legitimate authority. Such activities included the authorization of the transfer and discharge of patients, ordering of blood tests, determination of ideal dry weights for patients and determination of heparin dosages. All these tasks are outside the legal area of practice for nurses in Victoria, but nurses found that they had to initiate actions in these areas and seek out medical personal to sign covering orders.

Nurse-patient relationship

The nature of renal units, catering as they do for chronic patients and entailing a long-term, ongoing relationship with them, was seen by the participants as providing environments in which conflicts emerge between the nurse and the patient. These conflicts were recognized as a major source of dilemmas.

Establishing an initial relationship with patients was seen as 'very difficult'. Conflict arose between nurses and patients because the patients did not believe that the nurse had the expertise required to provide adequate care. The nurse had to 'prove' her skill before the patient would demonstrate trust in her. Over time, this conflict resolved, as the relationship shifted from 'distant' and 'distrustful' to that of friendship, which involved mutual support.

In spite of this, personal involvement with patients, an aspect inherent in the long-term relationship established between nurse and patient, created the potential for the development of dilemmas. Patients frequently vented their anger on nurses; anger at being on dialysis, anger at developing complications, anger at having to cope with changing family relationships. The dilemma for nurses was how to respond 'professionally' while being a 'friend'.

At times, nurses perceived patients as treating them poorly, demonstrating little respect for their knowledge and expertise. Many patients were described as demanding. Males, in particular, tried to dominate the nurse in their relationship. Some patients were described as being abusive and rude. Nurses viewed many patients as relating to them inappropriately and frequently found themselves in situations where they were angry at such treatment.

Nurse-nurse relationship

Nurses asserted that there were two types of dialysis nurses – those who 'just' came to work for their pay and the others who were involved in all levels of the unit operation. For the nurses who maintain a strong sense of personal commitment to dialysis nursing, the lack of similar commitment by their colleagues was frequently a source of dilemma. Avoiding participating in the resolution of problems outside the unit and avoiding overtime were cited as examples of a lack of commitment.

Conflict with nursing staff in other wards was an issue discussed by all the participants. The most frequently mentioned problems included ward staff using poor or incorrect procedures for peritoneal dialysis and technical problems with machines that were 'user initiated'. Ward staff were perceived by some nurses as inflexible and lacking organizational skills. The ward staff were described as not assessing the overall needs of the work situation; rather, they were seen as dealing with the immediate problems and doing the minimum amount of work.

Nurses who had more recently begun to work in the dialysis setting perceived many of the nurses with more dialysis experience as having poorer skills in relating to, and caring for, patients. They reported that some senior staff would use a technique of 'telling patients off' if they were doing things the senior nurse did not like. They saw some senior nurses as only assessing patients from the narrow perspective of renal dialysis, having lost the broader view of nursing the patient as involving many psychological and physical aspects. This is related by one nurse:

'Like if they are diabetic . . . they come in the morning and are unsteady on their feet, they [senior nurses] think immediately that they are dehydrated, they must be dry. And I say 'what about their blood glucose, have they had any breakfast?' They haven't thought about that. They are only directed toward dialysis, they don't see the rest.' (Ann)

Other nurses demonstrated less willingness to take responsibility for the more difficult aspects of patient care compared to nurses in senior positions. As one nurse said:

'I guess it really annoys me too, that it is left up to 'x' [a charge nurse] and me to go and tell patients when someone dies. None of the other staff will take that responsibility because they perceive that we [senior nurses] have had a lot of experience doing this.' (Julie)

Inter-nurse conflict, particularly amongst nurses in the dialysis unit, created feelings of anger and frustration.

Nurse-administration relationship

Nurses reported conflict in relationships with both nursing and general administration staff. Nursing administration was seen to interfere in the management of the unit at some levels and at other times was described as ignoring and being non-supportive of the dialysis staff.

The conflict between the ward and the renal unit nursing staff described above was one area where administration was seen to interfere unnecessarily. The nursing co-ordinator in one instance had offered to mediate between the ward and the dialysis unit. This 'over intervention' prohibited the ward and unit from resolving their own problems. The dialysis nurses saw administration as amplifying the problems rather than contributing to their resolution.

Another issue confronting nurses was the 'fight' for stores. Dialysers, blood lines and peritoneal dialysis equipment were cited as items that were frequently out of supply. These are items required to perform treatments and without which patients would be unable to dialyse.

Relative importance of conflicts

The importance of conflicts in relationships and the resultant dilemmas were not ordered by the frequency of their occurrence but by the degree to which the conflict restricted work. The degree and relative importance of the conflict varied according to the level of the nurse's dialysis experience. The less experienced nurse saw the nurse-patient relationship as the most significant source of dilemma, whereas the senior dialysis nurse identified the doctor-patient and doctor-nurse relationships as key. This difference in perspective is in part due to role demands on the senior nurse, who generally has more responsibility for overall service delivery and more experience with on-call and out of hours work.

The relative importance of the conflict in one relationship was influenced by the introduction of conflicts in other relationships and, in the view of the nurse, tended to shift the importance of some dilemmas. For example, dilemmas emerging from the conflict with medical staff or administration. There appeared to be a hierarchy of importance of dilemmas corresponding with the status of the person with whom, the conflict was being experienced – dilemmas with nurses being the least irritating, followed by patients, with medical and administration creating the greatest degree of conflict. The conflict between nurses was seen as frequently being personal. In these cases the nurses have blamed themselves for conflict that has emerged from the social setting in which they work. Several of the nurses apologised for criticising their peers.

Lack of control

Nurses identified a lack of control in determining patient care as a feature of the dilemmas experienced. Acute dialysis treatments graphically illustrated the lack of control experienced by these nurses. When dialysing patients with acute renal failure outside the dialysis unit environment, nurses described situations when they were left to maintain dialysis, using the telephone to consult with renal medical staff if concerns arose, after treatment was initiated.

One nurse described a situation where she had to seek senior medical intervention to stop dialysis treatment for a man with unstable blood pressure. It was only after three phone calls to medical staff that agreement to stop dialysis was obtained. The patient died shortly afterwards. She said:

'I just felt that we had put this person through all this trauma . . . and I just felt the powerlessness of nurses.' (Terri)

The lack of control over treatment while left alone to maintain it was identified as causing anxiety and stress for the nurse. In an attempt to gain control over

her practice, one nurse stated:

'Nurses are having almost like a power play continuously, because they are aware of things that doctors have authority over . . . the nurse really has to get strong if she cares enough about the treatment, and her own judgement, and value of self.' (Barbara)

Discussion

The findings of this study suggest that dilemmas encountered in dialysis nurse practice are related to the structure of the work environment. Understanding the role of the nurse in dialysis and the dilemmas encountered in practice may provide insight into the issues that nursing models for ethical practice could address.

Dialysis nurse role: a *de facto* medical role?

Nurses in this study perceived their role as more than an extension of medical care but were unable to articulate clearly the nature of that role, other than it being one of technical support. Much of the work of the dialysis nurses involved assuming a *de facto* medical role: ordering treatments and managing the more mundane aspects of the medical treatment of the dialysis patients. The nurse's role was predominantly one of a technical expert.

The data suggest that the notion of autonomy for these dialysis nurses is a belief rather than a reality. Many of the nurses stated that autonomy was the feature of their work that helped to keep them working in dialysis units. They perceived the work of nurses in wards as involving less autonomy that dialysis nursing. However, the description of their perception of the level of autonomy contradicts their description of the actual decision-making process in the work environment. Although they talked about autonomy, it is argued that they could not act as autonomous agents. Their actions required the approval of others, particularly medical staff.

The notion of autonomy, traditionally viewed as a central concept in nursing models (Evans 1986), seemed to have been adopted by the nurses in dialysis. The ideology of autonomy has been developed to account for their isolation and the *de facto* medical role they have assumed. Isolation from other nurses and workers in the institution has led dialysis nurses to believe that they are autonomous, but isolation did not equate with independent practice in the descriptions offered in this study. This false perception of autonomy by the dialysis nurse is crucial in developing an understanding of the dilemmas encountered in dialysis nurse practice.

Dilemmas emerging from conflicts

A lack of power to determine nursing action underlies the conflicts in relationships identified in this study. Dilemmas resulted from a lack of power over practice. These related to choice between the conflict of loyalties to other workers and to patients, choosing between the desire to maintain harmony in the work place and the maintenance of personal integrity. These dilemmas are seen essentially to be moral dilemmas, as they involve conflicting values.

These dilemmas are similar to those described by Rushton (1988) and Schaefer (1989). The dilemmas resulting from medical-nurse conflict confirm the medical dominance of the work environment of the nurses participating in this study as argued by Willis (1989). The three central concepts of autonomy, authority and sovereignty are present in the dialysis unit.

Medical autonomy has been shown where medical staff were able to manipulate the rules, and where registrars were able to decide their own practice without reference to others.

Medical authority was evident when nurses were unable to effect treatment changes without the approval of medical staff.

The sovereignty of doctors underpins the dilemmas involving patients. Patients demonstrated acceptance of doctors' control of their health when they failed to disclose openly their dissatisfaction with medical practice.

The analogy of the family (Game & Pringle 1983, Turner 1987) is also supported by the findings of this study. The dialysis nurse assumes the role of the 'wife'. She has a subservient role to that of the doctor and depends upon him both legally and 'practically' for her work. The doctor delegates the less desirable tasks of his role to the nurse. A paternalistic attitude by doctors and nurses toward patients was identified. This was evidenced in the attitude of some nurses in 'telling off' patients when they failed to do what the nurse required. The conflict between the junior and senior dialysis nurse relates in part to this paternalism, with the senior nurse seemingly accepting paternalism as part of her role and the junior nurse still wanting to challenge this relationship as unacceptable in practice.

Unresolved feelings

The unresolved feelings associated with dilemmas need to be addressed by the nurse to preserve her professional integrity. Further exploration of coping strategies employed in dialysis nursing will provide an opportunity for nurse administrators and educators to develop and promote positive and constructive means for dilemma resolution and for altering the environment so that the dilemmas do not emerge. Action research (Winter 1989) could be successfully employed within institutions to build supportive relationships between nursing administration and dialysis nurses while developing strategies that will assist nurses in gaining the power to structure nursing practice.

Further research directed at examination of the dilemmas encountered in other areas of nurse practice is suggested. This in turn could assist in developing curricula that will prepare nurses for the 'real' issues that emerge in practice, including conflicts and powerlessness encountered. The incorporation of these concepts will prepare nurses for the complexity of the work environment.

A limitation of this study was the use of only one data collection strategy, the open interview. The findings of this study could have been enhanced if observation had also been used to collect data. The size of the project and time constraints prohibited the use of secondary data collection strategies.

Conclusion

This study has indicated that dilemmas encountered in dialysis nurse practice are a direct outcome of conflicts in relationships within the work place. Conflict was found in relationships between medical staff and patients, medical staff and nurses, nurses and nurses, nurses and patients, and between nurses and administration staff.

Nurses have generated a belief regarding autonomy in practice that they have maintained despite the reality of their practice differing. Hence, an ideology of autonomy existed which sustained their practice by mystifying its reality. Problems are therefore individualized. Nurses do not address structural aspects of the environment in which they work.

The findings of this study challenge the use of current theoretical ethical frameworks to guide nursing practice. It is argued that these models need to be reexamined concerning the notion of nurse autonomy and acknowledgement of the medical dominance of the nurse's work environment. Given such acknowledgement, models can be developed which could enable nurses to increase their power over their practice, therefore assisting the effective positive resolution of such dilemmas.

Sally Wellard RN MN BA(SocSc) Renal Certificate Lecturer in Nursing, School of Nursing, Victoria College, Burwood Campus, Burwood Highway, Burwood, 3125, Victoria, Australia

References

Angus L.B. (1986) Research traditions, ideology and critical ethnography. *Discourse* 7(1), 61-67.

Davis A.J. & Aroskar M.A. (1978) *Ethical Dilemmas and Nursing Practice*. Appleton-Century-Crofts, New York.

Evans M. (1986) Not free to be moral. *The Australian Journal of Advanced Nursing* 11(3), 63-69.

Felton G.M. & Parsons M.A. (1987) The impact of nursing education on ethical/moral decision making. *Journal of Nursing Education* 26(1), 7-11.

Field P.A. & Morse J.M. (1985) *Nursing Research: The Application of Qualitative Approaches*. Croom Helm, London.

Fry S.T. (1989) Towards a theory of nursing ethics. Advances in *Nursing Science* 11(4), 9-22.

Game A. & Pringle R. (1983) *Gender at Work*. George Allen & Unwin, Sydney.

German C. (1986) Ethnography: the method. In *Nursing Research: A Qualitative Perspective* (Munhall P. & Oiler C. eds), Appelton-Century-Crofts, Norwalk, Connecticut.

Keats D. (1988) *Skilled Interviewing*. The Australian Council for Educational Research, Melbourne.

McClelland J.E. (1985) Report of the Committee of Enquiry into Nursing in Victoria vol. 1. Government Printing Office, Melbourne.

Muschamp D. (1989) Moral Dilemmas: What Are They and How Should Nurses Respond to Them? Nursing Law and Ethics, 2nd Victorian State Conference, Monash University: sponsored by Phillip Institute of Technology, School of Nursing, Bundoora, Victoria.

Opie A. (1989) Qualitative Methodology, Deconstructive Readings, Appropriation of the 'Other' and Empowerment. Paper presented at TASA Annual Conference, La Trobe University, Melbourne, 5-8 December.

Parse R.R., Coyne A.B. & Smith M.J. (1985) *Nursing Research: Qualitative Methods*. Brady Communications, Bowie, Maryland.

Richmond I.J. (`1986) Dialysis nurses coping with stress through a peer support group. *Journal of Nephrology Nursing* 3(22), 52-54.

Roberts S.J. (1983) Oppressed group behaviour: implications for nursing. *Advances in Nursing Science* 5(4), 21-30.

Rushton C.H. (1988) Ethical decision making in critical care: the role of the pediatric nurse. *Pediatric Nursing* 14(5), 411-412.

Sandelowski M. (1986) The problem of rigor in qualitative research. *Advances in Nursing Science* 8(3), 27-37.

Schaefer S. (1989) Patient advocacy: an ethical dilemma? *Focus on Critical Care* 16(3), 191-192.

Thompson I.E., Melia K.M. & Boyd K.M. (1983) *Nursing Ethics*. Churchill Livingstone, Edinburgh.

Turner B.S. (1987) *Medical Power and Social Knowledge*. Sage, London.

Willis E. (1989) *Medical Dominance* 2nd edn. Allen & Unwin, Sydney.

Winter R. (1989) *Learning from Experience: Principles and Practice in Action-Research*. Falmer Press, London.

RESOURCE 4

Tim Radford,
Guardian, July 29

Such a fine body of evidence

The world's leading physiologists gather in Britain next week to consider the eternal mystery of what it is to be human

What a piece of work is a man, said Hamlet, who didn't even have the advantage of an hour with Professor Denis Noble at Oxford University's physiology laboratory. Take for a moment the human heart. It beats for roughly 70 years at an average of 60 thumps per minute.

'And it manages that, in most cases, pretty faultlessly.' says Noble, who has spent most of his working life watching the cardiovascular system, and who next week will play host to 5,000 scientists at the 32nd congress in Glasgow of the International Union of Physiological Sciences, meeting in Britain for the first time since 1947.

'It's a phenomenal performance. No engineered pump ever manages anything remotely comparable to that. A really good athlete can get it down to close to 20 beats a minute. and the highest is about 200 per minute. Which means a really good athlete can increase the rate of flow of oxygen to the muscles by a factor of 10. That's a huge change in output.'

He thinks it is possible to imagine that one day science will make sense of the heart. It is a self-organising system. Although it is made up of four parts - two atria, two ventricles - in a sense there is only one heart muscle, because the several hundred million cells that make up the heart all talk to each other.

'Their excitation is connected together, so that once the pacemaker region of the heart sets the whole thing off, it spreads through the atria and into the ventricles on both sides, as though one is dealing with a unified structure. It is a marked example of a system in which co-operativity - the ability of cells to perform as an integrated whole - is of crucial importance, and with even a minor disturbance of that, you have trouble.'

The curious thing is that the heart is a piece of engineering with huge safety margins. Most people have four or five times as much heart muscle as they need: only superb athletes get close to using all of it. Suppose you have a heart attack: a massive one, which results in an infarct, or permanent damage to the heart muscle. If you survive the instant of attack, you can put up with the loss of 20 per cent of the heart tissue, and the heart goes on beating, despite the scarred muscle. The trick, for science, is not simply to understand what is happening in the cells, but in the organisation, the higher level of hierarchy, that makes up a whole heart.

Professor Noble thinks that one day science will solve the problem of the heart attack. The nervous system is something else. 'Think of the immensity of what we are trying to do. We are talking of a system that has 10 billion cells in it. Each of those has connections to another 1,000 maybe, so in terms of connections, we are talking about 10,000 billion; and there may even be information stored at a lower level than that, at the molecular level. This is like looking at a system that is at least as complex - in terms of total numbers of things to be looked at - as the universe itself. It would be utterly astonishing if we had got anywhere near understanding such a complex organ.'

In his work on the heart, he can imagine an endpoint: it may be 100 years hence, but it is conceivable. 'With the nervous system, that is totally inconceivable. This organ is, after all, the means with which we have generated our culture. Our culture has an aspect which is impossible for scientists to deal with, which is that it is history-dependent.'

Humans have what he calls 'intentionality' - what the Church used to call 'free will'. It is a characteristic of humans that they can choose to do things: they can choose to view themselves; an understanding of the nervous system would be inseparable from the choice to examine and understand it.

All that cannot be reduced to machinery. Professor Noble calls himself an arch anti-reductionist. When he says this, he is declaring sides in a quiet war going on in the biomedical sciences, between those who maintain that ultimately, humans are prisoners of their genes, and those who argue that they are not.

But then Professor Noble is used to taking sides. Seven years ago he and others founded an organisation called Save British Science, and since then has kicked the shins of successive cabinet ministers for their neglect of an important part of human culture. He is used to the notion of culture. When in the south of France he can pass as a Parisian, and he is one of the handful of Britons at home in Occitan, the old language of Languedoc, the tongue of the Troubadors. He plays the guitar and collects the songs of Gascony.

He insists, when in those countries, on delivering at least part of his lectures in Japanese and Korean. Congress delegates will be welcomed in 70 languages - including Occitan. When the encounter ends, he heads off to Oxford to buy a thicker brush to paint another welcome in Korean ideograms.

His argument against reducing humanity to the message of its genes has much to do with ideograms: the three Chinese characters for physiology stand separately for words that could also be translated as The Logic Of Life, the title of a book he has co-edited for the conference. He thinks it impossible to separate human physiology from the culture that makes us human. The seeming inability of the Chinese to digest milk products is only a matter of the precise stomach fauna created by their traditional cuisine which reinforces the cuisine culture. All land vertebrates have the same number of bones but the musculature is vastly different. The advantage to humans of being able to execute fine movements with their hands would have been one of the driving forces of evolution, and also of the development of the nervous system.

In that sense, the nervous system is dependent on human history, and the human culture that led to the ideograms for the logic of life, and it would be pretty hard to disentangle a gene for that. He speaks in a week in which there has been a furore about the discovery of a gene or genes for a predisposition to male homosexuality, but he sidesteps that issue and chooses a simpler example. Even the zebra's stripes present a problem of the logic of life.

'It is obviously not the case that there is a genetic code for each stripe. What must be programmed is the ability to form a pattern. There must be ways in which the system organises itself from fairly minimal programming of the information required to put it all together. In the whole of the genetic code, there cannot be all the information that is, at the moment, in our nervous systems. A lot must be left to the properties of self-organising systems which have got minimal coding to get them going. On that, we have a very long way to go.'

He also thinks that one of the things that alarms the public about science is simply the idea of the selfish gene: of the human as a vehicle for the survival of the genes and their passing on to another generation. 'I have turned that on its head. I am saying, no, that is wrong. Genes are not free-roving selfish individuals: they are prisoners of the successful physiological systems that carry them. Put that way, no one is frightened. I am not using biological information in a different way from the selfish gene material. I am putting it in a different way that respects the hierarchy or orders.'

So, he argues, it is implausible that humans should be able to understand themselves just by understanding the human genome. 'It is a bit like thinking that somebody who understands the machine code of a computer understands what the computer is doing.'

He chooses a text from Pascal as the theme of the conference: 'I find it impossible to understand the parts without understanding the whole, and to understand the whole without knowing the parts in detail.'

So the congress will have room for everybody: there exist so far 15 tons of printed paper, containing 3,000 abstracts of papers he has yet to examine. It is likely to touch on all the issues of what it is to be human: from the behaviour of the human physique in zero-gravity to the capacity of human divers to work at depths of up to 1,000 metres.

It will also tackle what he sees as one of the great problems facing modern man: his longevity. The heart - and most of the other human organs - have colossal safety margins simple because of human evolutionary history. Modern human life is the profoundest, wallowing luxury compared to the privations of most hominids through recent millions of years. Humans are adapted to survive in harsh conditions, and tend to expire from heart attacks brought on by sugar, fats, tobacco and alcohol.

'We are not really well adapted to being well off. Nor are we well adapted, most of us, to living to 80, because why should evolution worry about it? Apart from the evolutionary value of a few survivors to pass on the culture, it isn't obvious why the majority should have survived, and of course they didn't. The majority were dead by 30. Those who survived to 60 or 70 were very rare. Why are we complaining that, because we die of heart attacks at 65, we are badly off? By God, compared to our predecessors, we are doing very well indeed.'

Hamlet, on the other hand, died young, as did many of his contemporaries.

The Logic Of Life: The Challenge of Integrative Physiology, edited by C.A.R. Boyd and D. Noble (Oxford £8.95)

RESOURCE 5

Patricia Lyne, Biochemistry, Session Five – The power supply, The Open Learning Foundation ,1994

Mitochondria – cellular 'power stations'

Where mitochondria occur

Figure 1 on page 8 shows two specialised types of cell. Take another look at it now – you will see that each cell contains round or oval structures labelled mitochondria. These are sub-cellular structures concerned with the conversion of chemical energy derived from food into a form of energy which cells can use in all the kinds of work that they do.

Mitochondria occur in all living cells, and the more active the cell – the more work it has to do – the more mitochondria it will contain. Very active cells contain thousands of mitochondria.

They tend to accumulate in the parts of the cell where most activity takes place. For example, sperm are very active structures. They are sometimes referred to as 'naked nuclei', containing very little apart from the genetic material.

Figure 14 shows that, in fact, the sperm contains something else as well, to aid it as it moves towards the egg. It contains a stack of mitochondria arranged at the base of its tail, to provide the energy it needs in order to sustain movement as it travels towards the neck of the womb.

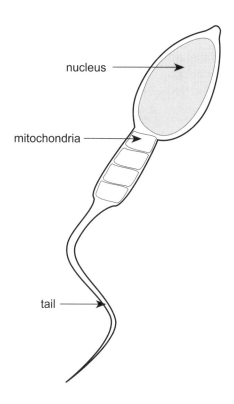

Figure 14 Diagram of a single human sperm

Mitochondria are also plentiful in all the specialised cells which we are using as examples in this unit. These are all very active, but in different ways. Muscle requires energy for movement and heat production. Pancreatic cells need energy for the synthesis of insulin, and intestinal epithelial cells need energy for active transport.

Young mammals, including human babies, have a specialised tissue called 'brown fat'. This is a form of fatty tissue which has a very high concentration of mitochondria arranged in such a way that the form of energy which emerges is heat. This tissue produces additional heat to assist the infant in withstanding cold conditions during the early days of its life, when it isn't mobile and therefore not producing a great deal of heat through muscular movement.

So we find mitochondria in all living cells, providing the form of energy which those cells need. But how did they get there in the first place? There are some interesting ideas about their origin, as we will see next.

The origins of mitochondria

The singular of mitochondria is **mitochondrion**. Unlike the other sub-cellular structures, each mitochondrion contains its own genetic information in the form of DNA, and can divide to produce two new mitochondria independently of the division of the nucleus.

During sexual reproduction, the egg contains mitochondria derived from the mother. The sperm also contains mitochondria, as you saw in *Figure 14*, but these don't survive in the egg after fertilisation. This means that mitochondria are transmitted through the female line only. Some scientists believe that mitochondrial DNA represents a direct link back to the first human females.

The origins of mitochondria lie further back in time than that, however. Because they have their own DNA and can grow and divide independently, many scientists believe that they originated as free-living, independent bacteria. Somehow, these took up residence inside living cells early in the history of life on earth. The arrangement proved beneficial to both parties, so the bacteria remained in the cells and developed into mitochondria as we know them today.

The structure of mitochondria

Mitochondria are larger than many of the sub-cellular structures such as ribosomes. They are just about visible when a living cell is viewed with the ordinary light microscope. In different cell types they vary in shape, size and numbers. When they are studied at very high magnification using an electron microscope, it can be seen that each mitochondrion has an outer and inner membrane boundary.

The inner one is folded inwards to produce a large surface area, rather like irregular shelves, inside the mitochondrion. At very high magnification, the shelves (**cristae**) are seen to contain batteries of enzymes arranged in regular patterns. Between the shelves lies the mitochondrial matrix, in which a further range of enzymes is located. *Figure 15* shows the structure of a mitochondrion as seen in an electron micrograph.

When tissues are prepared for electron microscopy they are sliced very thinly indeed. So the photographs which we see represent the cut surfaces of the structures through which each slice passes. *Figure 15* shows how an oval shaped mitochondrion looks if it is cut through lengthways.

From this brief description it should be clear that the inside of a mitochondrion is very highly organised.

Like everything in the human body, it is adapted to perform a particular task. This degree of organisation is required for efficient energy conversion, as we will see after the following brief summary.

Summary

- Usually the cells are supplied with plenty of oxygen by the blood.

- Under these circumstances, pyruvic acid and the hydrogen produced as a result of glycolysis enter the mitochondria.

- Mitochondria are sub-cellular structures found in all living cells.

- They are most plentiful where cells are undertaking intensive work.

- Mitochondria can move and divide independently of the nucleus. They contain DNA.

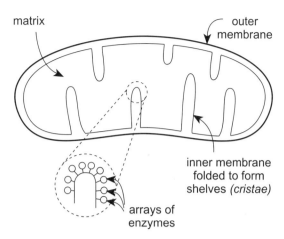

Figure 15 The structure of a mitochondrion

- For this reason, some scientists consider that they were originally free-living bacteria.

- Each mitochondrion is bounded by a double membrane. The inner one is folded into shelves (cristae) which produce a large internal surface area.

- The inside of the mitochondrion contains highly organised sets of enzymes.

What happens in the mitochondria?

Can you remember tracing the fate of glucose when it was being used as fuel in the absence of oxygen? We explained that this process gave a relatively small energy yield in the form of two molecules of ATP for each one of glucose.

The end products of this process, glycolysis, are pyruvic acid and hydrogen atoms. To liberate the energy which they contain in a useful form, they must enter the mitochondria.

They cross the mitochondrial membrane through specialised structures, which we could regard as the 'gates' to the mitochondrion in the same way that we have already visualised the 'glucose gates' into the cell. These gates only open if oxygen is present.

After pyruvic acid has passed through the gates, it undergoes a reaction to form a compound with just two carbon atoms. We'll call this the C_2 **acid**. The third carbon atom is converted into CO_2.

The C_2 acid first encounters a series of enzymes in the matrix. This series is called the **tricarboxylic acid cycle (TCA)** or sometimes the **Krebs' cycle**, after its discoverer.

This set of enzymes is found in all living cells, and represents one of the fundamental processes of life.

A brief outline of what happens goes something like this.

First, the C_2 acid combines with a C_4 acid to become a C_6 acid. This then undergoes a series of rearrangements, each catalysed by a different enzyme, in which:

- the original C_4 acid is reformed, ready to go round the cycle again

- the two carbons from the C_2 acid are converted to CO_2, and leave the cell as a waste product

- the energy from the chemical bonds in the C_2 acid is converted and handed on, with hydrogen atoms, to the final stage in the process which takes place on the cristae.

This process, together with glycolysis, is summarised in *Figure 16*.

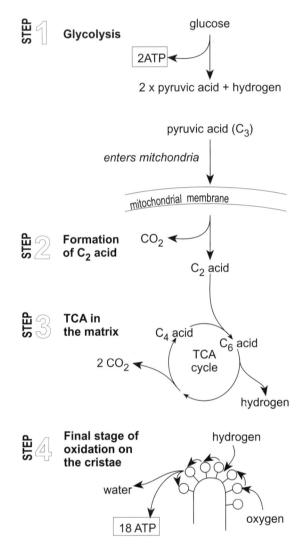

Figure 16 A summary of the complete breakdown of glucose

The final stage in the whole process occurs on the cristae when, through a further series of reactions, the hydrogen reacts with oxygen to produce water.

This is the stage when most of the energy is handed over to ADP, which has been formed during cellular work, and is ready to be recharged.

Eighteen ADP molecules are 'recharged' to ATP in the mitochondria for each molecule of pyruvic acid. However, each glucose molecule gives rise to two of pyruvic acid, so the total number of ATPs per glucose is 36 molecules through the TCA and two from glycolysis – a total of 38. It is not essential to remember these particular numbers, but it is important to notice the difference between the gain in ATP (two molecules) during glycolysis in the absence of oxygen, and the gain during complete oxidation of glucose through the TCA (38 molecules).

All the processes occurring in the mitochondria can be summarised by a third equation which shows what happens to the pyruvic acid. Instead of acting as a dump for the excess hydrogen, as in *Equation 2*, it is completely broken down to carbon dioxide.

Equation 3

$2 \times C_3H_4O_3 + \quad 4H \quad + 6O_2 + 36ADP + 36P \quad \rightarrow \quad 6CO_2 + 6H_2O + 36ATP$
(pyruvic acid) (hydrogen)   (enzymes
                                               of TCA)

ACTIVITY 35

This activity provides practice in answering equations.

First, check that *Equation 3* balances. Satisfy yourself that there are the same number of atoms on each side of the arrow. Are all the atoms which were present in the molecules of pyruvic acid accounted for?

Secondly, combine *Equations 1* and *3* together to give the overall summary equation for the breakdown of one glucose molecule. In other words, write down the two equations one after the other, and remove the intermediate stages.

For example, if our two equations looked like this:

A + B = C + D

and

C + D = X + Y

then writing the two together gives

A + B = C + D; C + D = X + Y

Therefore, we cancel the intermediate stage and say

A + B = X + Y

Your task is more complicated than this, but it is possible to combine the equations in a similar way, and discover that they still balance. It will be easier to do this if you leave out the ATP and write the equations like this.

Equation 1
$C_6H_{12}O_6$ $\rightarrow$ $2 \times C_3H_4O_3 + 4H$ [Gain = 2ATP]
(glucose)   (enzymes of   (pyruvic acid)
                glycolysis)

Equation 3
$2 \times C_3H_4O_3 + 4H + \quad 6O_2 \quad \rightarrow 6CO_2 + 6H_2O$ [Gain = 36 ATP]
(pyruvic acid)   (oxygen)   (enzymes
                          of TCA)

Commentary

Writing *Equations 1* and *3* together gives
$C_6H_{12}O_6 \rightarrow 2xC_3H_4O_3 + 4H$ [Gain = 2ATP]
             $2xC_3H_4O_3 + 4H + 6O_2 \rightarrow 6CO_2 + 6H_2O$ [Gain = 36 ATP]

Equation 4

$$C_6H_{12}O_6 + 6O_2 \rightarrow 6CO_2 + 6H_2O \qquad \text{[Gain 38 ATP]}$$

This last equation is the summary of the complete breakdown of glucose in the presence of oxygen – the complete oxidation of glucose.

This may already be familiar to you as it is often used, in simplified versions, to describe the fate of glucose inside living cells:

glucose + oxygen $\rightarrow$ carbon dioxide, water and energy

or $C_6H_{12}O_6 + 6O_2 \rightarrow 6CO_2 + 6H_2O + \text{energy}$

I have unpacked this simple equation because I wanted you to appreciate that it is a summary of a very complex and beautifully organised sequence of events that is happening at this moment in every cell of your body, and on which all life depends.

You may prefer to use the simplified version to summarise the sequence.

There is no need to remember the details of the other one, but I hope that it has given you an appreciation of what is really involved in this apparently simple process, which is usually called **tissue respiration**.

Efficiency and pollution

The requirements for a real power station are that it should convert energy to a useful form efficiently, with a minimum of waste products and with as little harmful pollution as possible.

The cell has the same requirements. When oxygen is present, there is a good yield of ATP for every molecule of glucose fuel used. Energy which is not 'captured' as ATP is liberated as heat, which is useful to maintain body temperature, so the overall process is efficient.

The waste products are water and carbon dioxide. The latter is the only harmful source of pollution, and requires a mechanism for its removal from the body. The water is an important internal source for the body and is either reused or removed into the bloodstream.

Summary

- In the mitochondria, pyruvic acid is completely oxidised to CO_2 and water.

- This occurs in two complex series of reactions.

- The first is the TCA cycle, carried out by enzymes in the mitochondrial matrix.

- The second takes place on the mitochondrial cristae. Here, the hydrogen and energy 'bundles' react with oxygen. During this process, the energy is channelled into ATP production.

- A total of 38 molecules of ATP are made overall during the oxidation of one glucose molecule, including the two produced during glycolysis.

- The overall equation for the oxidation of glucose, tissue respiration, is $C_6H_{12}O_6 \rightarrow 6CO_2 + 6H_2O$.

- This system is efficient and the only harmful waste product is CO_2.

- ADP is recharged, re-forming ATP, on the mitochondrial cristae.

● This process only occurs in the presence of oxygen.

● The main function of the mitochondria is to provide a constant supply of the energy source ATP.

Alternative fuels

Although glucose is the main fuel source for cells, and is the only source that brain cells normally use, other foods can also be used to produce ATP and so supply useful energy.

You may recall that proteins are broken down into their building blocks, the amino acids. These are mostly required to build cellular proteins; therefore they are too valuable to be used as fuel – using them in this way would be like burning your furniture to keep your house warm. However, the body has no way of storing amino acids so, if there's an excess, some of them will be converted into glucose or into the acids that take part in the TCA and will be channelled into the oxidative pathway described earlier.

Fats are a true alternative fuel supply. Indeed, they are the preferred supply for some types of muscle. They provide the basic materials for the construction of many cellular structures. Excess fats can be stored and readily converted into one of the intermediates in the chain of reactions through which pyruvic acid is oxidised. They thus feed into the process which produces ATP in the mitochondria. I will describe exactly how this happens when we discuss the integration of these metabolic pathways in the final session of this unit.

Fats are a very good fuel source for most cells, but if they are used exclusively a pollution problem can arise. In order for fats to enter the TCA some carbohydrate fuel must be used as well. We could say that if fats are to be used as fuel in the cellular power stations, a carbohydrate 'booster' is needed. If this is not available, by-products from fat oxidation pile up. These are compounds called **ketones** and they result from the incomplete 'burning' of fat in the absence of carbohydrate.

Nail polish remover contains a member of the ketone family – **acetone**. The ketones produced in the body have the same kind of smell as acetone, and this smell can be detected on the breath if ketones accumulate. This is not a problem in itself, but accumulated ketones are acidic and they reduce the pH of the blood plasma. This affects many parts of the body, including the brain. If uncorrected, progressive acidosis leads to coma and death.

A healthy person uses a mixture of the two main fuels under normal conditions and therefore has no problem with the accumulation of ketones. However, if food intake is restricted for any reason, the body will start to use up its fat reserves and the proportion of fat used as fuel will increase. Ketones start to accumulate.

In small amounts, these can be removed by an increase in the output of urine – they are 'washed out' of the blood. This usually happens when a person starts to lose weight by dieting. They may be detected in the urine by an appropriate test.

A person with untreated diabetes is unable to use carbohydrates within his or her cells, and is in the same position as someone who is starving. Their bodies will use their fat stores as fuel and ketones will accumulate. Large quantities of urine are passed because the body needs to get rid of the ketones. This results in thirst and dehydration. The classic early symptoms of diabetes mellitus are thirst, weight loss and a high output of urine, as we saw in Jason's case study in *Activity 23*.

ACTIVITY 36

Returning to the case study of Jason, this activity asks you to apply all the biochemical understanding you have achieved so far to this case.

First, read the following case study and review the relevant sessions of this unit. You could also read *Resource 1* and *Resource 5*, which provide additional background material. As you read these sources, consider the underlying biochemical events which are giving rise to the observed symptoms. After you've read the case study, write a short account – just a single paragraph – of these events.

Six months after his doctor's provisional diagnosis was confirmed, Jason is brought into the Accident and Emergency Department late one Friday evening. He had collapsed in the street outside a city-centre pub.

On arrival it looks as though he is just another heavy drinker, but a routine blood test shows a very high blood sugar level. He is deeply unconscious. He looks very undernourished, his eyes are deeply sunk in their sockets and his skin looks strange. When pinched, it doesn't quickly spring back to normal.

Jason's breathing is deep and rapid. He has obviously been drinking as he smells of beer, but there is another fruity smell too, as if he'd been mixing beer and sherry in quantity.

The friend who accompanies him tells the staff that he is a diabetic – a fact which Jason has only recently discovered. Apparently he doesn't talk about it a lot, so his friend doesn't know how he deals with his injections.

Now please write your short account of the biochemical events occurring in Jason's body.

Commentary

Jason could well have been mistaken for a drinker, but clearly his condition is related to his diabetes. Since his blood sugar is so high, it looks as if he has been neglecting to take his insulin.

The high blood sugar shows that his cells are not taking in glucose. It is not passing through the gates in the cell membranes, as described in Session Four. His body is therefore using fat as its main energy source, and ketones are accumulating as a result, giving rise to the fruity smell on his breath.

As the ketones have accumulated, the pH of his blood has fallen, affecting his rate of respiration and causing progressive unconsciousness.

Jason's body will have produced large amounts of urine to remove ketones and glucose from his blood. He is therefore dehydrated, as shown by his sunken eyes and inelastic skin.

Jason is going to need rehydration and the right amount of insulin to restore his blood sugar to normal, and to enable him to use glucose as a fuel in his cells. He is also going to need education and support when he is over this crisis, to help him to adjust to a problem which will be with him for life.

The episode we have just described is a **diabetic coma**, caused by a high concentration of sugar and ketones in the blood. Jason will have to learn to cope with the diabetic's other problem – too little blood sugar caused by an imbalance between insulin injected and carbohydrate in the diet. You can read how this affects a person in *Resource 5*.

Summary

- Both fats and proteins can be oxidised through the same metabolic pathway as carbohydrate.

- Since proteins are needed for other purposes, they are not normally used as a fuel supply.

- Fats are a major alternative to glucose as fuel supply.

- Oxidation of fat requires a carbohydrate 'booster'.

- If this is not available, fat oxidation results in the accumulation of harmful ketones.

- Diabetes mellitus results from a failure of insulin production.

- If insulin is not replaced in people with this condition, fat is oxidised, ketones accumulate and severe symptoms follow.

This concludes our study of the way that cells use fuels, derived from food, to produce useful energy for their work.

The hormone insulin has figured in this session, and will do so again in Session Six as we consider how proteins such as this are packaged by the cell for transport to the place where they will be used.

Asthma: a hidden disease of our times

RESOURCE 6

Andrew Nocon and Tim Booth, Nursing Standard, August 1/Volume 4/ Number 45/1990

Andrew Nocon and Tim Booth explore the impact of asthma on the sufferers' everyday lives and argue that nurses need to be more aware of its practical and emotional effects.

One in five children suffers from asthma at some time.

Asthma is a hidden disease. Few people are aware that one in five children suffer from the condition at some time (1), or that one in 15 adults also experience symptoms (2). Yet most people know someone with asthma, either in their own family or among their close acquaintances.

The popular image of asthma is of a mild form of wheezing. But it was not melodramatic for a recent episode of Casualty to show a young girl dying from a severe attack: deaths in England and Wales remain around 2,000 a year – and, if anything, are slightly increasing (3) – despite the availability of better medication and increasing diagnosis by doctors. All the signs are that it is becoming more widespread.

The development of new drugs has meant that many people are able to manage their condition effectively. But this does not mean that asthma can yet be cured or that sufferers can be relieved of all symptoms. Where symptoms persist, doctors frequently blame this on a failure by patients to comply with medical instructions, either in the prevention of symptoms or in handling attacks when they do occur. For some people, though, the available drugs simply do not succeed in providing adequate control.

Other people are able to relieve symptoms when they occur, though they cannot prevent them from arising in the first place. Some, especially those with very severe asthma, have to strike an uneasy balance between control of the condition itself and unpleasant side-effects from the medication. Many avoid the onset of symptoms by avoiding situations and activities which might trigger them off.

A study which we carried out recently in Sheffield shows that asthma can have a severe impact on the everyday lives of sufferers and their families. The study focused on the 'sharp' end: on people who had been admitted to hospital with asthma a year earlier. While some of these people experienced only mild or short-term effects on their lives, others were severely incapacitated.

John, Peter and Mary illustrate the problems that people face. While the details of their situations are unlikely to be replicated exactly by other sufferers, the overall extent to which asthma affected their everyday lives, including both its practical and its emotional impact, reflects the average for the people who took part in this study.

John is two years old. He has had asthma since the age of ten months. He typically starts to cough and wheeze when he catches a cold. Winter tends to be a bad time for him, especially as there is a problem of damp in the house. During the winter months, he might have symptoms for about a week at a time, then be free of them for another week or so before they come on again.

Preventive drugs

In addition to medication to relieve attacks, he also take regular preventive drugs. The medication sometimes gives him stomach-aches or makes him sick. He became extremely agitated when he was put on a course of oral steroids following a bad attack. A year ago, he was admitted to hospital for two days. His parents believe this admission would not have been necessary if the GP practice had not lent out it's last nebuliser.

John's parents were advised to get rid of their dog as animals often bring on attacks – though his parents do not believe this was a factor in his own case. They also replaced his feather pillows and duvet with synthetic ones – again, this does not appear to have helped. Nevertheless, his mother does additional dusting and cleaning in his room in order to reduce the dust that might set off his asthma.

In the past, both of John's parents lost time from work because of his condition. His mother in fact had to give up her job. Her sister had previously looked after him while she went out to work. But when his condition got worse, his aunt became worried that she would not know what to do if he had a bad attack. She felt unable to look after him.

In the early days, John's condition caused his parents many sleepless nights and a good deal of worry. The resultant strain, on top of other family problems, let to violent rows and brought them close to splitting up. While the strain is now reduced, John's asthma is still a source of much worry for his parents. They are concerned about the way that it may affect him as he grows older. Bad attacks are themselves very frightening, especially when he cannot breathe, starts to turn blue and needs urgent medical help.

Four-year-old Peter has just started school. His asthma started two years ago, two months after his father left home. Like John, symptoms often follow the onset of a cold but other factors also trigger them off, especially pollen, smoke and the smell of pigs or paint. They are also sparked off if he becomes upset or excited. During the past year his asthma has been under better control and the amount of drugs he takes has been reduced. Like John, he is on preventive medication as well as drugs for symptom relief. But he attends a different hospital from John and has been provided with a nebuliser.

Peter's asthma means that he cannot have the pets that he would now like. As in John's case, Peter's mother bought synthetic bedding to replace his feather duvet; but, for Peter, this change has definitely helped to prevent symptoms from occurring. She also makes a point of asking visitors not to smoke.

Peter himself sometimes has problems when he is out walking or if he takes part in sport at school – but his asthma does not prevent him from joining in. He does have to avoid bonfires – which means that he has to stay indoors on bonfire night. Even the smoke from candles on a birthday cake can trigger him off.

Peter's mother previously had to take time off work to look after him – and lost money as a result. Although she now has a part-time job, she still had to accompany him on a recent school trip and took along his nebuliser. For her, too, Peter's condition means extra housework. The asthma now only tends to worry her when he has a bad attack. Nevertheless, she continues to feel angry with her ex-husband for having contributed, however unwittingly, to its onset, with all the resultant suffering that it has caused him.

Social impact

Our study showed that the social impact of asthma was more marked for children below school age than for children at school. It was most severe of all, though, for adults. Mary's situation illustrates the problems that can arise. She is 55, and first developed asthma when she was 41, during a holiday. It is now triggered off by dust, grass, wool, fur, cold weather, the smell of paint, cooking vapours, personal worries, seeing other people wheeze, and even the sight of dust.

Mary has been in and out of hospital a good deal, though she has not had any further in-patient treatment since her last admission a year ago. Despite being on preventive medication, she suffers symptoms everyday – and the drugs for relieving them do not always work. She has had to cut down on some of the drugs anyway because they had an adverse effect on her blood-sugar level. They also affect her sight. Housework is a great problem for her. She cannot do any vacuuming or dusting, the steam from the iron can set off her asthma, and she has difficulty making the beds or doing any washing by hand.

Friendly advice

Like John and Peter, Mary replaced a feather pillow with a synthetic one, and benefited from the change. Unlike the two boys, though, the advice came not from a doctor but from a friend. And it was only after her own experience of fumes from a paraffin heater that she replaced it with an electric one.

Outside activities cause her problems. She cannot carry heavy shopping or do any gardening or decorating. Walking uphill is extremely difficult. In addition, she feels embarrassed using her inhaler in public. Mary said that the overall effect of the asthma was to make her feel old and decrepit.

Until a few years ago, she worked as a packer in a sweet factory but the dust from the sugar brought on attacks. When they were bad she used to go to the toilet and try to recover while her colleagues covered up for her. Eventually she was forced to give up. She is now very pessimistic about her chances of ever getting another job.

Although Mary has not had a severe attack for over a year, she is very worried that she could have another bad attack at any time. At present, she feels locked up inside her house and unable to lead a normal life. If she had more money, she would emigrate to Jamaica, her place of birth, where she does not suffer from asthma at all.

These case extracts illustrate some of the everyday ways that asthma affects individual sufferers. We have avoided the more sensational stories – though there were plenty of these among the 50 people interviewed: adults and children in intensive care units, cardiac failure resulting from asthma, the attempted suicide of a 30-year-old woman, the sterilisation of a woman of 24 following miscarriages due to asthma, and the decision of another 24-year-old woman not to marry her boyfriend in case her condition should get worse and he should feel obliged to look after her.

There are a number of ways in which nurses could help sufferers and their families. First, sufferers want more information about asthma. Many of the people we spoke to wanted to know more about the reasons they have attacks, and the point at which they should seek medical help.

Some parents of asthmatic children blamed themselves for its onset: they wondered whether it might have genetic causes or be due to difficulties during pregnancy. They had not had the opportunity to discuss these fears with medical or nursing staff.

Sufferers also wanted to know more about the drugs they had been prescribed and any side-effects these might have. Because of fears about possible long-term effects, some people were thinking of reducing the amount of drugs they took. They wanted to know what would happen if they did, and whether any alternative medication might be available.

Many of the respondents who did not have a home nebuliser said they very much wanted one. However, doctors seemed to vary in their opinions about home nebulisers: there are both pros and cons to the debate (4). Many sufferers wanted the opportunity to discuss this issue in more detail. Almost all the people we spoke to referred to the considerable emotional distress that asthma can cause. This was particularly true at the time of serious attacks. For many people, asthma led to longer-term emotional difficulties.

Some sufferers and relatives said they would have liked help to work through some of their anger, frustration, confusion, resentment, bitterness and sense of helplessness. They said counselling should be offered as a matter of course and not have to be sought.

Finally, several respondents spoke about their need for practical help. Housework and shopping caused particular difficulties. Some people could not use the bath without assistance. Others needed a telephone in order to summon help in an emergency.

A number of people did receive help from Social Services or the local asthma society. Many of them, though, had only found out about such organisations through friends or relatives. Other sufferers did not know what help might be available, or where to obtain it.

Nurses are well placed to help asthma sufferers and their families, either directly or by providing advice about services available elsewhere. It is essential, though, that professional staff should be aware of the wide range of problems that asthma can cause in people's everyday lives.

Andrew Nocon PhD, is a research associate at the Centre for Primary Care Research, University of Manchester. Tim Booth PhD, is director of the Joint Unit for Social Services Research, University of Sheffield.

References

1. Milner A.D. (1987) 'Recent advances in childhood asthma', Update, 34, 398-403.

2. Mortagy A.K., Howell J.B.L., Waters E.E. (1986) 'Respiratory symptoms and bronchial reactivity: identification of a syndrome and its relation to asthma', British Medical Journal, 293, 525-529.

3. Office of Population Censuses and Surveys (1988) OPCS Monitor: deaths by cause: 1987 registrations. DH2 88/3, London, OPCS.

4. Britton M. (1990) 'Are home nebulisers potentially dangerous?' MIMS Magazine, February, 69-75.

RESOURCE 7

Michael Surkitt-Parr, British Journal of Nursing, 1992, Vol 1, No 11

Hypothermia in surgical patients

During the perioperative period little attention is given to thermoregulation. This can lead to hypothermia which has severe physiological complications. This article discusses the causes and effects of hypothermia in surgical patients and describes a study that the author conducted to discover the level of awareness on the subject among operating department staff.

Hypothermia is a decrease in an individual's core temperature to 35°C or less (Flacke and Flacke, 1983). Hypothermia occurring during surgery is said to be inadvertent because it occurs accidentally in the absence of protective reflexes such as shivering. Although inadvertent hypothermia in the operating department was recognized in the 1880s as being the result of a cold environmental temperature (Lunn, 1969; Newman, 1971), it still appears to be largely overlooked in clinical practice.

Maintenance of the homeostatic mechanisms that regulate fluid and electrolyte balance is at the forefront of both medical and nursing practice during surgical intervention (Roe, 1973) and there is a wealth of literature on the subject. However, little attention appears to be paid to thermoregulation, an equally important homeostatic mechanism whereby body temperature is maintained within normal limits by balancing heat production and heat loss.

Heat is generated by the body by internal metabolism and from the external environment if this is higher than body temperature. Heat is also produced by body movement and by ingestion of hot food or liquid. Heat is constantly being lost to the environment through convection, radiation and conduction, through evaporation from the lungs and skin, and through urine and faeces. When heat loss is equal to heat production an individual is in heat balance, but when the two are not in equilibrium, body heat and consequently body temperature either increases or decreases.

Inadvertent hypothermia can readily occur in patients undergoing surgery when there is reduced heat production and a greater potential for heat loss to the environment. The major contributing factors are the withholding of oral intake preoperatively, diminished central nervous system (CNS) activity due to the administration of premedicant drugs and inactivity and unconsciousness resulting from the administration of a general anaesthetic. Spinal and epidural anaesthetics can also cause gross vasodilatation, leading to heat loss. In addition, patients undergoing surgery may have their skin prepared with cold and often volatile antiseptic agents and subsequently large body cavities may be opened.

Effects of hypothermia

A hypothermic patient can suffer cardiovascular, neurological, haematological, immunological and metabolic problems as well as disturbances in fluid and electrolyte balance. Cardiovascular effects may include atrial arrhythmias but at 30°C there is the possibility of spontaneous ventricular fibrillation (Reuler, 1978). Body temperature is also related to limb blood flow (Pflug *et al*, 1980). A decreased blood flow in the extremities has been associated with venous stasis which may precipitate vascular complications. Venous thrombosis has been documented in countries where surgery has been performed under cold conditions (Lunn, 1969) but virtually no such problems are encountered in warm, subtropical regions.

In hypothermia, cardiac output increases to help maintain adequate oxygenation, but this can soon lead to decreased output and ultimately metabolic acidosis. Hypothermia shifts the oxygen dissociation curve to the left, such that haemoglobin will have a greater affinity for oxygen and will not release this oxygen as readily at tissue level. This can result in tissue hypoxia with anaerobic metabolism and lactic acidosis (Vaughan *et al*, 1981). The majority of enzymes work most efficiently at 36.5-37°C, therefore all general metabolism will suffer with prolonged hypothermia. The neurological effects of inadvertent hypothermia consist of sluggish reactions and thought processes together with loss of coordination, but these are largely masked by general anaesthesia. However, they can make immediate postoperative neurological examination difficult.

Other effects include a decreased blood flow to the brain, diminished reflexes and dilated pupils (Rango, 1980). The immunological effects may result in decreased resistance to infection, but this could also be attributed to factors such as poor nutritional status (Roberts, 1979).

Hypothermia can also impair renal tubular secretion. Water, sodium and potassium are lost in greater amounts in the urine. This leads in turn to a rise in haematocrit (De Lapp, 1983). Low serum potassium can also cause cardiac arrhythmias and muscle weakness.

Factors that contribute to inadvertent hypothermia

Although there is an abundance of literature on inadvertent hypothermia in the operating department, there are few recent studies. However, many of the original findings are still relevant today. Research studies have identified a wide range of contributing factors: ambient operating room temperature (Goldberg and Roe, 1967; Morris and Wilkey, 1970; Morris, 1971), length of surgery (Goldberg and Roe, 1967; Babcock et al, 1979), age (Goldberg and Roe, 1967; Vaughan et al, 1981), and body type of patient (Babcock et al, 1979). They relate not only to the patient as a physiological being but also to the type of surgery and the environment (Closs et al, 1986).

Anaesthesia is the first scenario within the operating department for the patient, and its effects on the body, which render the patient unconscious, are major ones. It is possible that the development of inadvertent hypothermia may be related to the type of anaesthesia employed. General anaesthesia depresses the hypothermic thermoregulating centre. Skeletal muscle relaxants and CNS depressants abolish shivering and eliminate motor activity. Volatile anaesthetic agents are potent vasodilators and facilitate blood flow to the skin, thus contributing to heat loss through radiation and conduction (Fallacaro et al, 1986). Goldberg and Roe (1967) showed that the body temperature fell twice as much in patients given muscle relaxants as in those who had not received muscle relaxants. However, Morris (1971) found that the type of anaesthetic agent appears to have no significant effect on body temperature.

Stone et al (1981) studied the effects of heating and humidifying the anaesthetic gases and found that the greatest loss of heat occurs during the first hour of anaesthesia. This is supported by the work of Lombardi-Garner (1985) who found that 'heating and humidifying anaesthetic gases to 37°C and 100% relative humidity will effectively maintain the body temperatures of adults undergoing major surgical procedures under general anaesthesia'.

Once the patient is on the operating table a variety of preparatory procedures, which may have some thermoregulatory effect, are carried out. These include preparing the skin for surgery and positioning the patient, which often involve removing the patient's coverings for some time. Morris (1971) found that the greatest decrease in body temperature occurred during the first hour of anaesthesia. This was attributed to: exposure of a large area of skin before draping began; the use of skin preparations that caused heat loss by evaporation; and a large temperature gradient between the patient and the operating room. Wehmer and Baldwin (1986) showed that covering the patient with a warm blanket on arrival in the operating room, exposing only the skin over the operative site, and replacing the warm blanket immediately at the end of surgery 'protects the patient from the large patient to room temperature gradients that exist to keep the surgical team comfortable.' Also, the placing of a warming blanket under patients is useful during prolonged surgery.

The type of surgery and length of time on the operating table are relevant factors in the development of inadvertent hypothermia, but the effects of these factors are inconsistent. Neff (1987), when dealing with emergency trauma patients, found an increased incidence of hypothermia when thoracotomy and peritoneal lavage were being performed. The administration of cold intravenous fluids to the patient during the operation undoubtedly contributes further to a drop in body temperature. Babcock et al (1979) and Neff (1987) showed that the heat loss was related to the volume and rate of infusion. Heat loss was 70% greater when intra-abdominal surgery was being carried out and was further enhanced by the use of muscle relaxants and the subsequent decrease in heat production (Goldberg and Roe, 1967). In contrast, Morris (1971) found no evidence that heat loss was affected by the type of surgery (i.e. whether intra- or extra-abdominal).

Ideally the operating room temperature should be maintained at 21°C to ensure the comfort of patients and staff at all times. However, this temperature is not always achieved and the ambient operating room temperature has been shown to have the greatest effect on the incidence of inadvertent hypothermia.

In a study of operating room temperature, Morris (1971) showed that in '... rooms below 21°C all patients became hypothermic. At 21-24°C, 70% of patients remained normothermic and 30% became hypothermic. At 24-26°C all patients remained normothermic'. In this study the operative site, anaesthetic technique and age of the patient did not appear to significantly influence the effect of environmental temperature on the patient's body temperature.

Other studies (Goldberg and Roe, 1967; Morris, 1971; Babcock et al, 1979; Closs et al, 1986; Wehmer and Baldwin, 1986; Neff, 1987) have referred to ambient theatre temperature but have viewed it as a variable and not examined it specifically.

Goldberg and Roe (1967) negated gender as a causative factor in the incidence of hypothermia. However, they did show that the greater the age of the patient the greater the heat loss. Their study was undertaken in patients aged between 18 and 87 years: '. . . 78% of the patients studied experienced a temperature fall which was more pronounced in the elderly (>60 years)'. The reason given for this was that the reduced ability of the body to produce heat with increasing age incurred a heat deficit which led to a drop in temperature.

This is supported by Vaughan et al(1981) but discounted by Babcock et al (1979) who stated that body composition (amount of body fat) is also a relevant factor. Closs et al (1986) compared overweight and underweight patients and demonstrated that 'the greater the amount of body fat the smaller the fall in core temperature'. They further stated that 'age and ambient theatre temperature are highly significantly correlated with a reduction in core temperature' and concluded that body composition was a secondary contributory factor to patient age.

Table 1 Key factors in the development of inadvertent hypothermia

Not covering the patient with a warm blanket on arrival in theatre
Not heating and humidifying anaesthetic gases
Not restricting body exposure during skin preparation and positioning of patient
Length and type of surgery
Intravenous infusion of cold fluids
Ambient theatre temperature
Age of patient
Body composition of patient

The researcher was concerned about the level of staff awareness on the issue of inadvertent hypothermia as well as the possible incidence of hypothermia experienced by patients in the operating department. The main aim of this study was to determine operating department staff's awareness and understanding of the possible factors contributing to inadvertent hypothermia.

Methodology

The literature review identified a formidable list of key factors that contribute to the development of inadvertent hypothermia in the operating department (Table 1).

The two methodologies used were:

1. Participant observation: Observation records were developed for the reception area, anaesthetic room, operating theatre and recover room. Observations were made during specified periods varying from 30 minutes to two hours during daytime elective operating sessions.

2. Questionnaire to staff: The sample used in this part of the study were a group of 25 trained operating department nursing staff and operating department assistants (ODAs). No untrained staff were included as they always work under the direct supervision of a trained nurse or an ODA. The staff participating in the study comprised five ODAs, eight recovery room nurses and 12 theatre nurses. The length of theatre experience ranged from six months to 20 years. The theatre and recovery room nurses were either registered or enrolled nurses.

To overcome any weaknesses in the methodologies and to obtain as accurate a picture as possible with regard to inadvertent hypothermia, a process known as 'triangulation' was employed. Triangulation is the use of a combination of methodologies in a study of the same phenomenon (Denzin, 1978).

Analysis of findings

A number of points arose from the findings.

Transfer bay

This area seemed to be regarded purely as a thoroughfare for patients entering and leaving the department. The emphasis was very largely on aspects of patient safety, e.g. checking the patient's identity and ensuring that the consent form was signed.

No assessment was made of the patient's temperature and they were not asked if they felt warm enough. The fact that patients came to theatre on a trolley with a covering of just one sheet and blanket or on their bed with extra coverings would seem to indicate reliance on routine rather than assessing the needs of the patients individually.

Anaesthetic room

Patients are taken to the anaesthetic room as soon as they are checked into the department. In this area the patients are cared for by the ODA or nurse who checked them in.

Patients had the same amount of coverings on them in the anaesthetic room as they had on admission to the unit; if the patients came to theatre on their beds, then just one sheet and one blanket is placed on them when they are transferred onto an 'inside' theatre trolley. During the period of observation in the anaesthetic room, two patients were asked if they felt warm enough, which seemed to indicate an increase in patient-centred care. Only three respondents (12%) felt that patients were at risk of inadvertent hypothermia in the anaesthetic room, but 11 (44%) thought that the patient's temperature should be recorded there. This would appear to be a good area in which to establish a patient's base-line temperature.

Operating theatre

Twenty-four respondents (96%) felt that the operating theatre was the area in which the patient was at most risk of becoming hypothermic. Seventeen respondents (68%) thought that the temperature of the operating theatre was a likely contributing factor to the development of inadvertent hypothermia, thus supporting the view of Goldberg and Roe (1967). However, despite this, during the periods of observation no-one formally checked the operating theatre temperature, probably relying on how comfortable the environmental temperature felt to them, which can obviously be very different from the temperature of the patient. In addition, 21 respondents (84%) stated that length of surgery was a contributory factor, and nine (36%) thought it depended on whether or not the abdominal cavity was opened. The results of the questionnaire analysis showed the operating theatre to be an area of high risk for the patient to develop inadvertent hypothermia. In addition, 15 respondents (60%) felt that the patient's temperature should be recorded before commencement of surgery, 18 (72%) felt it should be recorded continuously during surgery, and 14 (56%) thought it should be recorded at the conclusion of surgery. Despite these responses, some of the practices seen during the observation period did not reflect this concern, with only 33% of patients being kept covered until skin preparation was ready to commence. However, in 83% of the observed patients the area of skin surface exposed was limited as far as possible. Immediately after operation more practical attempts were made to keep the patient warm in that all wet drapes were removed, and 50% of patients had a sheet applied at the conclusion of surgery. No patients had their temperatures recorded in theatre.

Recovery room

This was the final area to be considered. Fifty per cent of the observed patients were transferred from the operating table onto their beds which had been warmed during the period of their surgery. These patients also had more coverings on them than the 50% who were transferred onto recovery trolleys at the conclusion of surgery and were covered by the standard one sheet and one blanket. There was much more visible evidence of individualized nursing care in this area, possibly because the nurse:patient ratio was always 1:1. This may be why only five respondents (20%) felt that the recovery room was an area where the patient was at risk of inadvertent hypothermia. Although 19 respondents (76%) thought the patient's temperature should be recorded in this area, no patients had their temperature recorded, two patients were asked if they felt warm enough, and three patients were given extra blankets before their return journey to the ward - a time when 12 respondents (48%) felt the patient was at risk of becoming hypothermic.

Summary of results

The results of the data collection indicates that the staff's basic theoretical knowledge is quite good, in that the majority of respondents showed evidence of understanding the nature of inadvertent hypothermia and at what temperature it occurred.

The main factors identified in the literature as contributing to inadvertent hypothermia were largely supported by the staff in their responses to the questionnaire. These were: the ambient temperature of the operating theatre (Goldberg and Roe, 1967; Morris and Wilkey, 1970; Morris 1971), supported by 17 respondents (68%); the age of the patient (Goldberg and Roe, 1967; Vaughan et al (1981), supported by 18 respondents (72%); the length of surgery (Goldberg and Roe, 1967; Babcock et al, 1979), supported by 21 respondents (84%); and excessive exposure of the patient's skin (Morris, 1971; Wehmer and Baldwin, 1986), supported by a surprisingly low number of 5 respondents (20%). In the literature, the gender of the patient was shown not to be of relevance, and no respondents supported this factor. Nine respondents (36%) cited intra-abdominal surgery as a possible risk factor, but this was not shown to be a risk factor in the literature (Morris, 1971). The use of muscle relaxants was thought to be a relevant factor in the literature (Goldberg and Roe, 1967) but only two respondents (8%) supported this.

Conclusion

The overall aim of this study was achieved in that the level of theatre staff's awareness of inadvertent hypothermia as a potential patient problem was determined. The results of the questionnaire showed that the theatre staff had quite a high level of theoretical knowledge of this problem, but a raised awareness of it on a working basis was needed.

Points that should be considered for further study include: the difference in patient temperature regulation using traditional linen drapes as opposed to the water-repellent types; the change in patient's temperature during their journey from the ward to the theatre along corridors; and, finally, why inadvertent hypothermia is not given a higher profile as a patient problem by both medical and nursing staff.

This study identified gaps in our knowledge of inadvertent hypothermia which suggest that further research is needed in order that the condition can be detected and prevented.

Key points

● Hypothermia frequently occurs during surgery but little attention is paid to thermoregulation during surgical intervention.

● Hypothermic patients suffer cardiovascular, neurological, haematological, immunological and metabolic problems, as well as disturbances in fluid and electrolyte balance.

● Factors that contribute towards hypothermia in surgical patients include anaesthesia, ambient operating room temperature, length of surgery, age, body type, type of surgery, and intravenous infusion of cold fluids.

● The results of this study show that staff have a good understanding of the theory related to hypothermia during surgery, but need to be more aware of prevention in practice.

● Anaesthesia is the first scenario within the operating department for the patient, and its effects on the body, which render the patient unconscious, are major ones.

● Goldberg and Roe (1966) negated gender as a causative factor in the incidence of hypothermia. However, they did show that the greater the age of the patient the greater the heat loss.

● Twenty-four respondents (96%) felt that the operating theatre was the area in which the patient was at most risk of becoming hypothermic.

Mr Surkitt-Parr is Theatre Manager at Leicester General Hospital and is presently on secondment as Project Manager for Clinical Audit at the Leicester General Hospital, Gwendolen Road, Leicester.

References

Babcock L, Chung A, Black H, O'Hara V S (1979) Hypothermia during routine surgical procedures. Milit Med 144: 487-9

Closs S J, Macdonald I A, Hawthorn P J (1986) Factors affecting peri-operative body temperature J Adv Nurs 11(6): 739-44

De Lapp T D (1983) Accidental hypothermia. Am J Nurs 83(1): 63-67

Denzin N (1978) The Research Act. 2nd edn. McGraw Hill, New York

Fallacaro M D, Fallacaro N A, Radel T J (1986) Inadvertent hypothermia; etiology, effects and prevention. AORN J 44(1): 54-7, 60-61

Flacke J W, Flacke W E (1983) Inadvertent hypothermia; frequent, insidious and often serious. Semin Anaesth 2: 183

Goldberg M J, Roe C F (1967) Temperature changes during anaesthesia and operations. Arch Surg 93: 365-9

Lombardi-Garner C (1985) The effects of the heating and humidifying of anaesthetic gases on the maintenance of body temperature. AANA J 53(6): 473-76

Lunn M F (1969) Observations on heat gain and loss in surgery. Guys Hospital Reports 188: 117-27

Morris R H, Wilkey B R (1970) The effects of ambient temperature on patient temperature during surgery not involving body cavities. Anesthesiology 32: 102-7

Morris R H (1971) Operating room temperature and the anaesthetised paralysed patient. Arch Surg 102: 95-7

Neff J (1987) Hypothermia in emergency trauma centre patients. Emerg Nurs 13(6): 382

Newman B J (1971) Control of accidental hypothermia: occurrence and prevention of accidental hypothermia during vascular surgery. Anaesthesia 26: 177-87

Pflug A E, Foster C, Martin R W, Winter P M (1980) Limb blood flow: the influence of temperature during halothane-nitrous oxide anaesthesia. Arch Surg 115: 616-21

Rango N (1980) Old and cold: hypothermia in the elderly. Geriatrics 35: 93-6

Reuler J B (1978) Hypothermia: Pathophysiology, clinical settings, and management. Ann Intern Med 89: 519-27

Roberts N J (1979) Temperature and host defense. Microbiol Rev 43: 241-59

Roe C F (1973) Temperature regulation and energy metabolism in surgical patients. Prog Surg 12: 96-127

Stone D R, Downs J B, Paul W L, Perkins H M (1981) Adult body temperature and heated humidification of anaes-thetic gases during general anaesthesia. Anesth Analg 60: 736-41

Vaughan M S, Vaughan R W, Cord R C (1981) Postoperative hypothermia in adults: relationship of age, anaesthesia and shivering to rewarming. Anesth Analg 60: 746-51

Wehmer M A, Baldwin B J (1986) Inadvertent hypothermia. AORN J 44: 5

Killer cocktail addicts

RESOURCE 8

Christopher Long, Observer, Sunday 14 November 1993

Heavy exposure to the body's potent survival chemistry could provoke war crimes, says Christopher Long

You are reading this on a quiet Sunday in a leafy suburb. Suddenly there is a devastating bang. Instantly, your autonomic nervous system activates at peak performance.

A releasing factor, corticotrophin, acts on the pituitary gland in your brain, triggering the adrenal glands above your kidneys and your body is flooded with adrenalin, noradrenalin and cortisol.

Blood diverts from your stomach and skin, engorging your instantaneously turbo-charged brain, heart, lungs and limbs. A little later, naturally produced opiate painkillers, endorphins, add to the cocktail.

Your elbows clamp to protect your chest. Your head ducks, protectively. Your legs, in tension, kick the table. This topples a coffee pot falling at an accelerating speed of 32 feet per second/per second.

You decide you are not in immediate danger because the bang was caused by a child's firework. Your left hand moves sideways to catch the pot before it hits the floor.

The whole process has taken milliseconds, endowing the body with colossal strength and speed of reaction. Soon afterwards, you feel cold because of the diversion of blood from body surfaces and you might want a cigarette and a drink to calm your nerves – to return your system to 'normal'.

It is one of the most remarkable phenomena known to science and, because we do not use this complex electrical and chemical process very often, its potency as a survival system is normally devastatingly effective.

But, in Bosnia, millions of civilians, gunmen, journalists, United Nations peacekeepers and aid workers experience these effects hour by hour and sometimes minute by minute over periods of many months.

It is not unreasonable to suppose that there must be side effects to abnormal exposure to such intensely potent chemistry.

'It's more than likely,' says Christopher Mathias, Professor of Neurovascular Medicine at the University of London. 'It's something which we haven't studied enough. If possible, we should really be observing the before-and-after effects of this sort of stress.'

The most perplexing and distressing characteristic of the Balkan conflicts has been the gratuitous cruelty accompanying the racial purging and persecution of civilians. Frequently this takes the form of frenzied sexual atrocities, mutilations and orgiastic killing.

These obscenities are usually committed while the perpetrators are experiencing the effects of severe long-term, high-adrenalin stress and while under the conflicting 'upper' and 'downer' influences of alcohol and marijuana.

Many men in the war zones discover that sexual desire, and certainly sexual performance, deteriorate rapidly under sustained stress – in marked contrast to the experience of many women. Could massive chemical imbalances in the body be inducing men to perform ever greater excesses in a bid to stimulate their dulled senses to some semblance of normality?

'This could be the case,' says Mathias. 'We know that drugs and alcohol alone may stimulate desire but damage performance. But add them to the cocktail of chemistry created by intense stress and you've got a mess.

'We don't know what long-term high-intensity stress might bring. One theory is that it would cause hypertension, leading to potential heart attacks, strokes and kidney failure.'

Such predictions have been borne out by medical observations in Sarajevo. Furthermore, if the whole system is on alert all the time, the receptor regulation controlling the heart and blood vessels can 'down-regulate', meaning that when you withdrew the stimulus they underperform. Equally, continuous stress can cause the autonomic nerves, which control the entire response system, to malfunction. This might even lead to lethargy, dulling of the senses, feeling faint, which would only be enhanced by the endemic use of more alcohol and marijuana to 'calm the nerves' or 'feel better'.

The consequent likelihood of irrational perception, thinking and decision-making by soldiers, civilians, peace-keepers and observers becomes obvious. And, just as alcoholics and drug abusers may need another fix merely to feel 'normal' and bodies over-compensate or under-compensate for chemical imbalances, so people exposed to long-term stress and danger in war zones may need ever greater excesses of physical or sexual aggression in order that their senses and responses feel anything like normal.

Could all this explain, in part, the incidence of rape, sexual assault, physical torture and cruelty that seem endemic in Bosnia and Croatia?

'Sexual activity might indeed need higher levels of mental, sensual stimulation to induce physical responses,' Mathias says. 'This would particularly be the case if the brain's receptors have malfunctioned by extreme exposure to stress and danger. Young men could be deeply disturbed, either consciously or subconsciously, by these baffling effects.''

The nature of the Balkan conflicts may assist the process. In this unusual civil war with no clearly defined front lines, where danger exists everywhere, all the time, and victims in one valley are aggressors in the next, there is no refuge. Old friends and neighbours can be new enemies and aggressors at any moment. Irrational, arbitrary snipers operate anywhere, any time. No one ever relaxes. But the body's 'fear and flight' mechanisms were never designed for this.

'The long-term effects? My prognosis is that the peripheral organs like the heart, lungs, liver and kidneys will adapt to peace sooner than the brain,' Professor Mathias maintains. 'Unfortunately we just don't know enough about this to predict the long-term price of the mental effects on people who've lived through all this. We really need to know more about it.'
Christopher Long has been a front-line correspondent in former Yugoslavia since the conflicts began.

RESOURCE 9A

*Sue Barr,
Nursing Standard,
March 10/Volume 7/
Number 25/1993*

Managing pain in children – myths in practice

Sue Burr highlights some of the myths which prevent good practice in the management of children's pain.

That pain results in a crying child, is a cultural myth based on ignorance. It is more accurate to say that such a myth results in children experiencing pain unnecessarily.

Whether physical or psychological in nature, pain is a common and distressing experience of childhood, particularly for children who are ill and subjected to frightening and painful procedures, and who may be separated from family and home – all that is comforting and familiar.

Why then has little attention been given to this common experience? One reason is society's failure to view their needs as different from those of adults. The result has been that the major portion of work associated with this issue is focused on adults.

Research on children undergoing bone marrow aspiration suggests that the level of pain experienced by those under five years of age is five to ten times greater than that of the older child. This shatters the myth that young children do not feel pain as much as older children, let alone adults. The lack of research with children has inhibited the work of those wishing to take this issue forward.

Interpreting a child's cry

Fifty per cent of children in hospital are under five years of age and their verbal skills, the commonest way in which adults communicate, are limited. How then can a child communicate pain? Most people assume that a child cries or screams when in pain, and that a quiet child cannot be in pain; or they may assume that crying is caused by hunger or psychological distress, but such assumptions are dangerous.

Pain assessment tools are now being devised, used, evaluated and refined more frequently, but these are all based on behavioural changes, a common indicator of pain. Knowledge of a child's behaviour at each developmental stage is essential if deviations are to be identified. In addition, their personalities have to be considered, some being rather quiet and shy while others are noisy and extrovert. Parents or the child's main care giver are the best source of information. They can describe how their child copes with pain and the measurers taken to alleviate it. Too often their contribution is ignored. Initiatives enabling them to be partners in the assessment of pain, planning and administering therapeutic measures and evaluating their effectiveness, are being developed. But unfortunately, too many children continue to experience pain.

Doctors and nurses have the greatest power to initiate and implement change but too often this issue is not adequately addressed in educational programmes for health care professionals and many remain ignorant on the subject.

The Royal College of Nursing's Society of Paediatric Nursing decided to work towards putting 'pain in childhood' on the agenda of all those concerned with the care of children in health care settings, and to encourage nurses to share and develop their own knowledge and practice.

In addition, the Joint British Advisory Committee on Children's Nursing, which has representatives from medical, nursing and voluntary organisations, and of which both Action for Sick Children and the RCN's Society of Paediatric Nursing are members, agreed that each organisation

would highlight the need to give more attention to the subject.

Failing to gain support

In recent years there has been an upsurge of articles in both professional journals as well as those for general public readership. Exciting initiatives such as the development and use of pain assessment tools, patient controlled analgesia, diversional therapy and establishment of pain control teams are rapidly becoming more common. But many of these developments occur in regional paediatric units, whereas most children are nursed in their local hospital. Too often paediatric nurses fail to gain support from colleagues who lack knowledge of the recent developments in the prevention and alleviation of children's pain.

Research shows that fear of the 'needle' is such that children will deny pain to avoid injections, yet they continue to experience pain unnecessarily by the outdated practice of routine intramuscular injections given pre- and post-operatively. Please help destroy the myths and thus ensure a better quality of care for children.

Sue Burr MA, BA, RSCN, RGN, RHV, RNT is Royal College of Nursing Adviser in Paediatric Nursing.

References

1. Volpe J. Neurology of the Newborn Philadelphia, W.B. Saunders. 1981.

2. Haslam D. Age and the perception of pain. Psychosom. 1969. 15, 86.

3. Porter J, Jick H. Addiction rare in patients treated with narcotics. New Eng

Table 1 Pain in childhood	Source: Nursing 1987, 3, 24, 890.
Myths	**Facts**
Infants cannot feel pain because of an immature nervous system	Complete myelination not necessary for pain to be felt (1)
Children do not feel pain as much as adults	Tolerance to pain increases with age (2)
Narcotics cause respiratory depression and addiction	Narcotics are not more dangerous for children than for adults (3)
Active children are not in pain	Increased activity is frequently a sign of pain (4)
Sleeping children cannot be in pain	Pain may result in exhausted sleep (5)
A child engaged in play activities cannot be in pain	Children can use play as a diversion and coping mechanism (6)
Children always tell the truth about pain	Children may not admit to pain for fear of the 'needle' or being ignored (4)
Injections are not painful	62 per cent of hospital children (4-10 years) say injection is the 'worst hurt they have ever had' (4)
The nurse who gives the needle only receives negative feedback	Analgesia administration does not have to involve painful injections

Journal of Medicine. 1980. 302, 2, 123.

4. Eland J. The child who is hurting. Semin Oncol Nurs. 1985. 1, 2, 116-122.

5. Hawley D. Postoperative pain in children: Misconceptions, descriptions and interventions. Ped. Nurs. 1984. 10, 20-23.

6. McCaffery M. Nursing Management of the Patient with Pain. Philadelphia J.B. Lippencott. 1979.

RESOURCE 9B

Pauline Shelley

Managing pain in children – taking action

Pauline Shelley outlines some of the initiatives taken by Action for Sick Children to tackle the problems of children and pain.

Action for Sick Children has become increasingly concerned about the myths that surround children and pain. These range from the extraordinary belief that children feel little pain because they are small, to unsubstantiated fears that pain killers may harm them. The Royal College of Surgeons report, Pain After Surgery, published in 1990, confirmed widespread under-treatment of children's pain and many studies since have confirmed their conclusions.*

It is good nursing practice for children's nurses to work in partnership with parents, using the parents' special knowledge of their own child. In the case of pain, parents often instinctively recognise their child's problem, but accept the professionals' view that children feel less pain or will be damaged by strong analgesia. If doctors and nurses are confused about pain in children they are in danger of undermining parent's instincts about their own child.

'They didn't believe me'

Enlightened professionals accept that pain is what the person feeling it says it is. It is alarming, therefore, to hear how many children report that their feelings have been ignored. Even older, articulate children experience this problem. Twelve-year-old Daniel told us: 'At first they didn't believe me when I got the pain. They told me I was a fusspot.' Daniel had several months of painful treatment to replace a bone in a diseased hip and he and his parents were led to believe that pain was inevitable and had to be endured.

William, aged 14, had a spinal tumour. He told us that in the five weeks that it took to diagnose him he suffered intense, unalleviated pain. It was not until he was transferred to Great Ormond Street Hospital and came to the attention of the pain control team that he was given appropriate and real pain relief.

To help children and parents, Action for Sick Children published a leaflet in June 1992, entitled Children and Pain. We were fortunate in being given financial assistance by the Calouste Gulbenkian Foundation – strong supporters of children's rights – and in being able to commission Dr Priscilla Alderson to write it, as her own research had brought her into contact with children and families who were having difficulty in obtaining pain relief.

Children and Pain helps parents to understand that children feel pain just as adults do and that, under proper supervision, they can be given stronger pain relief than paracetamol. It discusses the use of different drugs and explains how children can be helped psychologically by stroking, rocking, cuddling, telling stories, listening to music and relaxation techniques. A page for children answers any questions they may have and offers a pain chart to help them describe their level of pain intensity.

We hope the pamphlet will encourage parents to feel confident in their knowledge of their own child, to use it to help the child through painful procedures, and enable them to speak out when they are unhappy about inadequate pain relief.

Our message is also that they should work closely with nurses. One of our intentions is to help reinforce the increasing numbers of paediatric professionals who are concerned that children's pain needs are not being met. By giving them a useful and practical tool to use on the ward, we hope to encourage the development of pain relief policies in their unit.

Contact person is needed

We consulted with more than 30 leading paediatric nurses, doctors, anaesthetists and psychologists to help us in drafting the leaflet. We asked them who parents should contact if they are not satisfied with the pain control their child is receiving in hospital. Not one of them could answer the question, thus highlighting the duty of managers to ensure that there is a named person responsible for children's pain relief and that there are

protocols for dealing with pain to which all staff subscribe.
Pauline Shelley is Information Officer, Action for Sick Children

Further Information

Children and Pain is available from Action for Sick Children, Argyle House, 29-31 Euston Road, London NW1 2SD. Price £1 for individual copies, 10 copies £7.50, 50 copies £30.

A list of references is available from Action for Sick Children Library – send 50p and a stamped addressed envelope.

RESOURCE 9C

Peter Jaffe

Managing pain in children – 'relief only when desperate'

Pain relief is poor management, argues Peter Jaffe. Pain control policies for children should focus on pain prevention.

Pain relief relies on reactive treatment; pain prevention should be the goal.

A parent writes to tell us of a child's experiences with pain following surgery. 'In May 1991, Mark had a bone operation and was given a painkilling injection in the recovery room. That day and the next, he received only Calpol to alleviate the pain. For the next three days he received relief only when desperate. Our request for regular pain relief was met with 'He needs to be more occupied.' It was a terrible time, lasting six days.

'A couple of months ago, Mark had a similar operation. This time, he was given an injection in the recovery room, followed by pain relief two hours later on the ward. Pethidine was given on a regular basis and after about three days, he needed only paracetamol. He had a slight breakthrough pain and it was much less distressing for him and for us.'

Prevention is the target

The difference between the two visits was the institution of a pain prevention policy. Pain relief is poor management and relies on reacting when things are already bad. Studies show that children receive 10 per cent of the pain relief that adults do for the same procedure, and nurses often do not give even this small quantity when prescribed; 25 per cent of children having cardiac surgery were given no relief at all.

Developing a pain prevention policy is often straightforward, as senior nursing and medical staff are less likely to believe that the stronger analgesics are dangerous or habit forming in children or babies. An effective policy requires senior staff to:

- Agree protocols for their juniors for regular relief after surgery
- Consider patient-controlled infusion pumps even in young children
- Do not wait to recognise pain or for the patient to ask
- Believe children when they say it hurts
- Plan ahead for procedures in wards, outpatient and A&E departments
- Remember children often do not cry when in pain but go still and quiet.

Painful procedures such as inserting chest drains and drips should be planned for, even in small babies. Few have lignocaine infiltration before drainage procedures, but stress hormone levels show that it hurts them just as much as adults. EMLA cream can offer relief, and has eased drip and venepuncture procedures. When attending clinic, children with diabetes will be found to have lower blood sugars if mothers apply the cream before the children leave home. Surprisingly, many diabetic children worry about hospital blood-taking.

Short anaesthesia or ketamine is often used in young children for lumbar punctures and bone marrows, especially when needed regularly, as in leukaemia. These and other permanent indwelling cannulae, for example Hickman lines or Portocaths, have transformed the fear.

In summary:

- Plan ahead for pain
- Administer adequate doses of analgesics
- Use infusion pumps where available
- Never ignore the patient's complaints.

Peter Jaffe FRCP is Consultant Paediatrician, Hillingdon Hospital, Uxbridge, Middlesex.

RESOURCE 9D

Noelle Llewellyn

Managing pain in children – APS: a multi-disciplinary team

Noelle Llewellyn discusses the structure and developing role of a paediatric acute pain service.

In 1990, the Hospitals for Sick Children, London, established a Paediatric Acute Pain Service (APS) to address the pain management needs of children undergoing surgery; the care of those with acute non-surgical pain; and those with chronic pain problems. The team's structure was based on recommendations in a Royal College of Surgeons and College of Anaesthetists report (1).Developing a service is an exciting and challenging time, but it must be handled with care, and establishing effective working relationships with the ward, theatre and anaesthetic department staff is crucial.

The objectives of the APS clinical nurse specialist were to establish the pain assessment and management practices used in the hospitals and to identify ways in which nursing and medical staff felt that improvements could be made. The main areas of activity for the APS team were identified as clinical service, development, training and education and research.

Round the clock service

The APS provides a 24-hour service; nursing staff work from nine to five, Monday to Friday, while the consultant anaesthetists combine the work of the APS with regular anaesthetic commitments. Out-of-hours service is provided by the duty anaesthetist. Its aim is to provide a proactive service, reducing the likelihood of a child receiving inadequate analgesia and the need to call on the duty anaesthetist.

All the pain service children are seen twice daily. The morning ward round is a time for planning and changing regimes where appropriate, and the afternoon ward round assesses the effectiveness of any changes and ensures that the duty anaesthetist is updated for the night. Clinical management involves seeing children preoperatively whenever possible, discussing analgesic options with the child and family, and education, when necessary.

The final decision about the analgesic technique used rests with the anaesthetist, but the wishes of child and family are always considered. Nursing staff are available during the day for advice or to intervene should analgesia be inadequate or adverse effects occur.

The development of our service has enabled the safe use of high technology analgesic techniques in general ward areas as well as the high dependency units (2).

Audit is an integral part of managing pain service patients, it includes evaluating quality and assessing the incidence and severity of side effects. A postoperative pain management standard, nursing practice guidelines (3, 4) and core care plans have been introduced to give nurses clear guidelines on their role and responsibilities. Nurse education involves teaching in the school of nursing, and participation at local and national study days (5), and turnover of ward staff necessitates an ongoing education programme. The APS is also involved in training medical staff.

More research is required in paediatric pain assessment and management, and the APS has recently appointed a research sister to undertake a one-year study into the management of postoperative pain. We have not yet attempted to show a correlation between the children with whom we are involved and a reduced stay in hospital, but children, families, and hospital staff have responded favourably to the team's efforts. A multidisciplinary approach to the management of pain is vital (6).

Although a paediatric acute pain service may not be feasible in some smaller units, the principles of a team approach to develop clinical skills, audit the service, participate in paid education and undertake research, may be applied to improve pain management and patient satisfaction.

Noelle Llewellyn SRN, RSCN, DPSN is Clinical Nurse Specialist, Acute Pain Service, The Hospitals for Sick Children, Great Ormond Street, London

References

1. Royal College of Surgeons of England and College of Anaesthetists. Pain After Surgery. London, RCS. 1990.

2. Bromage P. A postoperative pain management service. Anaesthesiology. 1988, 69, 3, 435-6.

3. Lyall J. Painful admission. Nursing Times. 1992, 88, 48, 44-6.

4. Lloyd-Thomas A, Howard R. Postoperative pain control in children. British Med Journal. 1992, 304, 6835, 1174-5.

5. Carr E. Pain-free states. Nursing Times. 1992, 88, 48, 44-6.

6. Hunter, D. Relief through teamwork. Nursing Times. 1991, 87, 17, 35-38.

Managing pain in children – Balanced analgesia for children

RESOURCE 9E

Neil Morton

Modern principles of pharmacology can lead to better analgesia with fewer side effects for children. Neil Morton explains why.

The principles of modern pharmacological pain management aim to anticipate and prevent pain whenever possible (pre-emptive analgesia); and to target drugs at several parts of the pain pathways at the same time (balanced analgesia).

Their application often allows lower doses of analgesics to be used, produces better analgesia with fewer side effects, and may reduce morbidity and hospital stay.

Pre-emptive analgesia: An increasing body of evidence from basic research and clinical studies suggests that giving analgesic drugs prior to the noxious stimulus reduces the effects of that stimulus. Lower amounts of pain mediators such as prostaglandins are produced from the wounded tissue and the hormone response to injury is reduced. This lessens the tendency for tissue breakdown in response to injury (catabolism).

Balanced analgesia: The painful stimulus produces local changes in the tissues and activates local pain receptors (nociceptors). These in turn send signals by small fast-conducting nerves to the spinal cord and then onwards to the brain. The brain then initiates marked hormonal and behavioural responses designed to limit the noxious stimulus and to help repair tissue damage. However, these same responses produce high circulating blood levels of catecholamines (eg. adrenaline, noradrenaline), cortisol and glucose. The catecholamines produce vasoconstriction in the peripheral tissues, in the pulmonary circulation and in organs such as the kidneys. Tachycardia and hypertension are also produced which increase oxygen demand and cardiac work. The intracranial pressure may rise and this may be significant in the head-injured patient or the very premature infant who is particularly

at risk of intraventricular haemorrhage. These babies also have particular problems with high blood glucose levels, as glucose spills over into the urine producing an osmotic diuresis, dehydration and a hyperosmolar state.

The aim of balanced analgesia is to block or modify the pain pathway, simultaneously, at seven points. This will reduce the amplification effect of a local tissue injury, producing effects on all the body's tissues via the hormonal response to injury.

The drugs used to achieve these aims are:
- Local anaesthetics eg EMLA cream, amethocaine drops, bupivacaine
- Opioides eg morphine
- Non-steroidal anti-inflammatory drugs (NSAIDS), eg diclofenac or ketorolac
- Paracetamol
- The intravenous and inhalational general anaesthetics.

Table 1 Surface anaesthesia		
Agent	**Formulation**	**Proven uses**
EMLA	Cream	Venepuncture
		Venous cannulation
		Prepucial adhesions
		Surface lesions
		Lumbar puncture
		Skin grafts
Amethocaine	Gel	Ditto
	Liposomal	Venepuncture
	Drops	Squint surgery
Lignocaine	Gel/ointment	Urethral catheterisation
	Spray	Circumcision
		Circumcision
		Endotracheal intubation

Local anaesthetic techniques

Surface anaesthesia: (*Table 1*) The skin is readily anaesthetised with EMLA cream (Astra Pharmaceuticals Ltd) applied at least one hour ahead of time under an occlusive dressing (eg Opsite, Tegaderm). Venepuncture or venous cannulation can

Fig. 1 The monitoring protocol for children receiving intravenous morphine infusions. The infusion rate is adjusted depending on the results of the hourly recordings. This protocol is easily adapted for children receiving subcutaneous morphine, patient-controlled morphine or for children undergoing sedation for investigative procedures.

Intravenous Morphine Infusion
(Please place completed chart in case notes)

Name......... Unit No ... DoB .... Age ...... Weight ...
Operation .... Date .....
Morphine concn. Img/kg in 50mls 0.9% Saline) ...
Rate from ...mis/hr to .... mis hr
Any adjustments (specify type, reason and time made) ......
Record hourly

Time	$So0_2$	Resp Rate	Sedation score	Pain score	Nausea score	Rate of infusion (mis/hr)	Volume left in syringe
			Eyes Open 0 = Spontaneously 1 = To speech 2 = To shake 3 = Unrousable (call doctor)	0 = No pain A = Asleep 1 = Not really sore 2 = Quite sore 3 = Very sore (Crying) (call doctor)	0 = None 1 = Nausea only 2 = Vomiting x 1 in last hour 3 = Vomiting>1 in last hour (call doctor)		

Call doctor if severe pain (score 3), patient unrousable (sedation score 3), $Sp0_2<90$ Respiration rate less than 10 if over 5 years, less than 20 if under 5 years, excessive nausea or vomiting, drip blocked/tissued or pump alarming.

Contact duty anaesthetist bleep 2602 if help needed, or Dr .... Home No ....

then be performed painlessly in most children. Small surface lesions can be excised under EMLA cream cover alone.

Alternatively, EMLA cream can be used to prepare the skin prior to infiltration of local anaesthetic around such lesions. If this is done by slowly injecting warmed local anaesthetic solution via a fine needle almost no stinging discomfort occurs.

EMLA cream has also been used for the division of prepucial adhesions, prior to lumbar puncture, prior to myringotomy, for preparation of the skin over the sites of vascular access reservoirs (eg Portacath), capillary blood samples, arterial lines and donor split skin grafts.

The addition of glyceryl trinitrate (GTN) to EMLA improves venous access as EMLA alone can cause vasoconstriction. Alternatives to EMLA are being researched to speed the onset of action. The most promising is amethocaine in either a gel or a liposome encapsulated formulation.

Interestingly, amethocaine drops have been used for surface anaesthesia of the conjunctiva after squint surgery in children. This provides excellent early analgesia, eliminating the need for stronger opioid analgesics and reducing the incidence of postoperative nausea.

Lignocaine gel, ointment or spray may be used to provide analgesia after circumcision and can be repeatedly applied.

Wound instillation and infiltration: The local instillation or infiltration of wounds with bupivacaine solution is remarkably effective for procedures such as heriotomy or pyloromyotomy.

Peripheral nerve blockade: (*Table 2*) Several hours of excellent postoperative analgesia can be provided by specific peripheral nerve blocks with plain (non-adrenaline-containing) solutions of bupivacaine, 0.25 or 0.5 per cent, up to a maximum of 2mg/kg.

Regional blockade: Larger areas can be anaesthetised by blocking nerve plexuses. The axillary approach to the brachial plexus is the easiest in children and gives analgesia of the whole upper limb. The lower limb is most readily anaesthetised by an iliacus fascia approach to the lumbosacral plexus.

Epidural techniques can be used in children, the caudal route being the most common approach. Single doses give long-lasting analgesia which can be extended if a catheter is placed in the epidural space and top-ups or continuous infusions are given. Spinal anaesthesia can also be used and has found a place for anaesthesia of premature and ex-premature babies who are in need of hernia repair.

Table 2 Peripheral nerve blockade

Block	Commonest uses
Penile block	Circumcision, meatotomy, division of prepucial adhesions
Ring block of digits	Toenail surgery, lacerations
Metacarpal block	Hand surgery
Metatarsal block	Foot surgery
Great auricular nerve block	Correction of prominent ears
Dental blocks	Extractions, orthodontics
Intercostal block	Thoracotomy, laparotomy, renal surgery
Femoral nerve block	Fractured shaft of femur
Inguinal block	Herniotomy, orchidopexy
Lateral cutaneous nerve of thigh	Skin graft donor site
Siatic block	Lower limb surgery

Opioid techniques

Morphine is still the gold standard for opioid analgesia. It can be given orally (eg MST) for chronic pain therapy, intramuscularly (IM), subcutaneously, intravenously, epidurally and intrathecally. The subcutaneous and intravenous routes can be used for patient-controlled analgesia in suitably selected school age children.

Healthy babies, more than three months of age, handle morphine the same as adults. In neonates, however, the duration of action is prolonged and the central nervous system of newborns is probably more sensitive to its effects. Suitable dosage regimes are shown in *Table 3*, but the key to safety is proper monitoring of all children receiving opioid infusions (*Fig. 1*).

The monitoring protocol should include regular hourly assessments of efficacy of analgesia, adverse effects, if any, and checks on the infusion system. Pain assessment can be difficult, but a simple four-point score can be applied.

Monitoring sedation levels is a good safety check; measuring respiratory rate and oxygen saturation will help detect morphine overdose. An apnoea monitor can be useful in neonates and infants below the age of six months.

Dosages are for guidance only and need to be titrated and adjusted on the basis of monitoring results to achieve optimal analgesia with the minimum of adverse effects.

Non-steroidal anti-inflammatory drugs (NSAIDS): These drugs hold great promise as pre-emptive analgesics and for incorporating in balanced analgesic regimes. They are prostaglandin inhibitors and reduce the local tissue response to injury.

Diclofenac is most readily given to children as a suppository because the IM formulation is extremely painful.

Ketorolac is much less painful by IM injection but can be given IV safely. Much lower doses of opioids can be used with regular administration of the above, and a suitable paediatric oral formulation of these agents is urgently required. Clinical trials of short-term perioperative use have not substantiated concerns about excessive bleeding and adverse renal effects.

Paracetamol: This is the most commonly used simple analgesic and there are many suitable paediatric formulations. Its mode of action is not yet fully understood but it is effective for mild to moderate dis-

comfort, particularly when used in combination with local anaesthetic techniques.

General anaesthesia: Most children having anything other than minor surgery will have a general anaesthetic and the agents used have an important role in reducing the response to surgery.

This is the case during major surgery; they will often have sedation continued for some time afterwards to minimise anxiety and pain in the Intensive Care Unit.

Conclusion: Combining a general anaesthetic, with an appropriate local anaesthetic technique, and a non-steroidal anti-inflammatory drug, with or without opioids, provides excellent analgesia for children of all ages. Anticipating and pre-empting pain requires lower doses of drugs, thereby reducing their adverse side effects.

Regular assessment of pain and monitoring for adverse effects allows modification of these techniques for all children including neonates and the critically ill.

Table 3 Opioid techniques	
Intravenous morphine	
Concentration 1 mg/kg in 50 mls	
Bolus dose 0.1-0.2 mg/kg	
Infusion rate age 0-1m:	5 µg/kg/h
1<3m:	10 µg/kg/h
>3m:	20 µg/kg/h
Subcutaneous morphine	
Concentration 1mg/kg in 20 mls	
Bolus dose 0.1-0.2 mg/kg	
Infusion rate age 0-1m:	5 µg/kg/h
1<3m:	10 µg/kg/h
>3m:	20 µg/kg/h
Patient controlled analgesia	
Concentration 1 mg/kg in 50 mls	
Bolus dose 20 µg/kg	
Lockout interval 5 minutes	
Background infusion nil	

Neil S Morton MD, ChB, FRCA, is Consultant in Paediatric Anaesthesia and Intensive Care, Royal Hospital for Sick Children, Glasgow.

Bibliography

Freeman J. A., *et al* Topical anaesthesia of the skin: a review. *Paediatric Anaesthesia.*

Gillespie J.A., Morton N.S. Patient controlled analgesia for children: a review. *Paediatric Anaesthesia* .1992. 2, 51-59.

Lloyd-Thomas A. R. Pain management in paediatric patients. *British Journal of Anaesthesia.* 1990, 64, 85-103.

Morton N.S. Development of a monitoring protocal for safe use of opioids in children.

Paediatric Anaesthesia. In press.

RESOURCE 9F

Richard Lansdown

Managing pain in Children – playing monsters and dragons

Richard Lansdown explores some psychological approaches that help children to manage their own experiences with pain.

'This hospital is a holiday camp.' said one mother whose child would be undergoing a procedure that would involve pain. 'But it is a holiday camp with needles.'

We, as carers, cannot get away from the needles, or the other sources of pain, but psychological management can help. First we need to be sure that the child is aware that something is going to hurt; those who have been warned are able to cope more effectively than those for whom the experience is a shock. They key is to be realistic and matter of fact, and to time the information appropriately; children will often tell you how much notice they would like.

Survival aspects of pain

The second question is more complex, relating to the child's perception of the cause of the pain. The younger the child, the more likely he or she will be to think in concrete terms; pain is nasty and occurs because someone has done something wrong. Some children – authorities vary on the proportion – see their illness, and therefore their pain, as a punishment. While one must not assume that all young children have the same perception, it is worth checking on. As they get older they can see that pain can have survival value: a headache, for example, can give messages that medical attention is required and it can be mental as well as physical.

This leads to further questioning: are we dealing with a one-off pain, for example a pre-med, or are we considering the problems of repeated invasive procedures?

Are we looking at the chronic pain of cancer or migraine? Dealing with each is likely to be different. One overall rule, no matter what coping technique is used, is to give children permission to express their feelings, as long as this does not interfere with treatment: 'Yell as much as you like – but keep still.' One child was given a whistle to blow when the needle hurt, a strategy that proved helpful for him.

A rule of thumb is that distraction techniques are to be tried first for the one-off, here today and gone tomorrow experiences. Bubble blowing is often used, with bubbles blown from a metal rod dipped into soapy water. This methods works better when the children are active.

Rather than simply telling children that you want them to watch the bubbles, it is better to have them participate, so that they blow the bubbles themselves or count them, or see how far they can go. Story telling, if there is a book with pictures, and especially a book with pop-up pictures for younger children, can be of great help.

Children should become engrossed in the distracting activity before the painful procedure begins, and so it is important to have staff co-operation. Needless to say, this approach should not be used within a framework of tricking the child; there is always the need to give warning of impending discomfort.

Encouraging children to go to imaginary places where there is no pain and everyone is having a good time can be helpful for repeated injections or chronic pain. Once again, it is vital to try to bring the child into the action. We may think that imagining being in a quiet country village with warm sunshine lying round a rose garden will be calming but children often prefer images of monsters and dragons.

Some children accept that there is going to be pain; they cope by reframing the circumstance in which they experience it. A teenage boy who was having lumbar punctures pretended he was a spy, captured by the enemy who were torturing him. If he kept quiet that signified that he had not given away any of his comrades.

Hypnosis is now used in a number of hospital settings and has been shown to be of value with children as young as five years of age. The process is usually straightforward, but it is not without its dangers and should be used with supervision.

We can help in many ways; and if one technique is unsuccessful, we can try another. Hospitals will never be holiday camps but we can achieve much to avoid some of the dread associated with them.

Richard Lansdown PhD, FBPsS, CPsychol is Consultant Psychologist, The Hospitals for Sick Children, Great Ormond Street, London.

Managing pain in children – pain scales for toddlers

RESOURCE 9G

Sylvia Buckingham

Sylvia Buckingham outlines the issues involved and the problems experienced when devising a pain assessment tool for toddlers who had undergone day case surgery.

Assessing pain in children has always been a challenging area for paediatric nurses (1-4). Toddlers are at a vital stage of development, one in which their perceptions and understanding change rapidly, but they are also at a disadvantage in having a limited vocabulary and experience of communicating with the wider world. It is paramount, however, that nurses provide good communication and appropriate explanations if they are to develop a relationship with toddlers and their families (5, 6).

Paediatric nurses require information specific to the age group for whom they are caring, as in the case of the toddler who has specific developmental needs. And North American nurses have written prolifically about the development of pain assessment tools (4, 6, 7).

Patient assessment is fundamental to nursing action and is the linchpin on which subsequent nursing care hangs; yet, discussions undertaken over a period of several years show that no pain assessment tool has been implemented. Why then do we not use them?

Most tools require the child's participation and rely on his or her understanding of numbers, colours or drawings, as well as an ability to communicate verbally, to be able to see and to be alert enough to respond. Hence it can be argued that many of the pain assessment tools are invalid when used with toddlers.

Identifying behaviours

In 1990, I undertook a study to attempt to develop criteria which could be used as a basis for assessing toddlers for pain (8). A triangulated research-design approach was used to gain information from different perspectives : semi-structured interviews, questionnaires and participant observation. An initial analysis of the data identified both positive and negative behaviours of toddlers who were in pain following surgery (*Table 1*). The positive behaviours indicate that the toddler is not in pain, the negative that he or she is feeling pain.

The data also revealed less easily classified behavioural responses, or influencing factors:

- Absence/presence of main carer
- Accessibility of child to enable vital signs to be taken without disruption
- Disruptive presence of nurse (seeing a nurse could make a toddler anxious/cry)
- Inability of toddler to communicate effectively due to age, illness, medication
- Ability of aids to daily living needs obscuring pain behaviours
- Limited knowledge of 'normal' behaviour for that child
- Nurses' knowledge of type of illness/pain; type of premedication given and effect; type of analgesia prescribed and effect
- Nurses' ability to set appropriate 'ground rules' with the main carer
- Nurses' understanding of pain behaviours in the toddler.

These factors were then incorporated into a pain assessment tool.

The absence of the main carer can influence the behaviour of the toddler but a comprehensive paediatric nursing assessment of the situation using the tool, and a knowledge of the influencing factors, can assess whether the toddler is in pain and requires analgesia. This should form the basis of the assessment which should be repeated every 30 minutes to one hour, depending on the results.

Assessing vital signs

The research identified the need for paediatric training for nurses caring for children in pain, as subtle cues did not appear to be easily recognised by non-paediatric staff. Nurses' pain assessment skills were, not surprisingly, related to the child's behaviour and the nurses' ability to use visual observation and listening skills; identifying normal behaviour patterns (for that child and in general); assessing vital signs when other factors made these of limited value; implementing the concept of shared care; and knowledge of analgesia.

Behavioural cues from toddlers are often subtle and difficult to pick up in a busy ward where nurses may have several children to care for. Relying on parents may not always be possible and if they are to help, then the ground rules must be made clear or misunderstandings could arise (7, 9).

Using a behaviour indicator for pain assessment should be introduced to children and parents before it is needed to help their understanding of how it will work and what will be expected of them.

One of the major hurdles is the inconsistency of medical staff in prescribing post operative analgesia. Ideally they should be involved in the development of pain assessment criteria for it to be fully implemented. Ultimately, however, the crux of the problem may lie with nurses.

We must change the way we think about pain. It is something almost everyone experiences, regardless of age or illness, and it must be discussed with our patients and families before it happens.

Until we change our attitude to pain and pain assessment and make it an overt part of nursing practice we may forever be seeking the answer to treating patients in pain.

Sylvia Buckingham RSCN, DipN(Lond), BEd(Hons), RNT, is Head of Paediatric Nursing, King's College Hospital, London.

References

1. Hurley A, Whelan E. Cognitive development and children's perception of pain. Paediatric Pain. 1984, 14, 1, 21-24.

2. Kline J. Recovery room care for the child in pain. Maternal Child Nursing. 1984, 9, 261-264.

3. Holm K, Cohen F et al. Effect of personal pain experience on pain assessment. Image. Journal of Nursing Scholarship. 1989. 21, 2, 72-75.

4. McGrath P. Pain in Children. London, Guildford Press. 1990.

5. Douthit J. Patient care guidelines. Psychological assessment and management of paediatric pain. Journal of Emergency Nursing. 1990. 16, 3, 168-171.

6. Davis K. L. Postoperative pain in toddlers, nurses' assessment and intervention. In Tyler D, Drane E. (eds). Advances in Pain Research and Therapy. Paediatric Pain. New York, Raven Press. 1990.

7. Eland J. M. Children's pain. Developmentally appropriate methods to improve identification of source, intensity and relevant intervening variables. In Felton G, Albert M. (eds) Nursing Research: A monograph for Non Nursing Researchers. Boston, Littlejohn. 1985.

8. Buckingham S. An Exploratory Investigation into How Nurses Use Their Skills and Knowledge to Assess Postoperative Daycase Toddlers For Pain. London, University of the South Bank. 1991. Unpublished dissertation.

9. Copp L. A. Perspectives on Pain. Edinburgh, Churchill Livingstone. 1985.

Table 1 Behaviours.

POSITIVE	NEGATIVE
Verbal communication	
Chatting to carer	Unresponsive
	Says 'Ow'
	Crying
	Screaming
	Grizzling
Facial expression	
Looks happy/relaxed	Sad
	Unhappy
	Miserable
Body language	
Relaxed	Drawing up knees
Sitting on lap	Curled into ball
Active	Touches area that hurts
Cuddling	Unable/afraid to cuddle
Interested in surroundings	Stiff/holding area
Playing	Anxious/upset
Sleeping	

(Playing and sleeping are two behaviours which require further analysis to ensure that the toddler is not in pain. Vigorous play can camouflage quite severe pain and feigned sleep or superficial sleep can identify the toddler who has given up on complaining)

Physiological changes	
TRP and BP within normal range	Elevated TPR and BP
The toddler with chronic pain may have normal responses	
Activities of daily living (ADL)	
Drinks and settles	Drinks, remains unsettled
Eats and settles	Vomits
Passes urine and settles	Passes urine, remains unsettled

Managing pain in children – special care for special babies

RESOURCE 9H

Margaret Sparshott

Newborns may show different responses to acute, extreme, and chronic or long lasting pain. Margaret Sparshott discusses the role of nurses in providing treatment and comfort.

The experiences of sick newborn and pre-term infants in special care baby units are inevitably traumatic: to keep such babies alive, many invasive procedures have to be carried out. On the other hand, the late gestational and newborn periods are times of intense development of the cerebral cortex, so that an appropriate environment is essential for the newborn to ensure symmetrical development of the neurological system.

Babies are capable of experiencing pain from at least 30 weeks gestational age, and probably before (1). This experience is not subjective, however, since a baby cannot distinguish between what is painful and what causes discomfort.

Newborn babies show they are in pain by behavioural responses and physiological changes. There are certain types of cry (2, 3, 4), facial expressions (5), and body movements (6) that are associated with pain sensation. These responses are not available to fragile or pre-term infants, but in these cases, changes in heart rate, respiration, blood pressure, skin and toe temperature and blood oxygenation can indicate stress from any cause (7, 8).

Changes in the endocrine system (1), and an increase in palmar sweating (9) are also indications of pain in the newborn, but these signs are of no practical value to nurses undertaking bedside care.

Responses to pain

The infant may show different responses to acute, extreme, and chronic or long lasting pain. In the case of extreme pain, crying and grimacing are accompanied by axial stiffening, head extension, and an abnormal position of the limbs. The infant in chronic pain may not cry, but appear inert and unresponsive, showing diminished communication with the outside world, and even an expression of hostility (10). Acute pain is felt during and following invasive procedures such as heel-prick sampling, lumbar puncture, or insertion of intravenous cannulae. Good techniques in carrying out such procedures help to mitigate and limit suffering, and a baby can often be comforted by cuddling, swaddling, and nutritive or non-nutritive sucking.

Babies suffering from painful illnesses such as necrotising enterocolitis or meningitis cannot be consoled in this way. The cause of extreme pain must be relieved and appropriate analgesia administered. Analgesia will also be necessary for the infant suffering from chronic pain: the most common are morphine sulphate, paracetamol and nerve blocks such as lignocaine (11).

A nursing care plan for managing pain in the newborn may be a useful guide to demonstrate the effect pain has on the patient (11). This plan should include:

- The problems of pain from traumatic procedures, post-surgery, and illness
- The goals: prevention of unnecessary suffering: maintenance of a safe environment; restoring a state of equilibrium
- The nursing interventions available to achieve these goals.

Since what is perceived as uncomfortable by one baby may be experienced as painful by another, the world of the newborn in hospital should be made free from all forms of distraction and discomfort. For example, controlling light and noise levels, and alleviating the problems posed by separation from parents.

Listing categories of environmental disturbance and appropriate interventions will guide nurses in choosing the most effective method of consolation or treatment for each baby (12). And, of course, they should use their own knowledge and experience of the infants in their care to find appropriate ways to comfort and stimulate.

Margaret Sparshott RGN, RM, is a staff nurse in the Special Care Baby Unit, Plymouth General Hospital.

References

1. Anand K, Hickey P. Pain and its effects in the newborn neonate and fetus. The New England Journal of Medicine. 1987. 317, 21, 1321-9.

2. Bowlby J. Attachment. London, Pelican Books. 1969.

3. Michelsson R, Jarvenpaa A *et al.* Sound spectrographic analysis of pain cry in preterm infants. Early Human Development. 1983. 8, 141-9.

4. Wolke D. Environmental and developmental neonatology. Journal of Reproductive and Infant Psychology. 1987. 5, 1, 7-42.

5. Grunau R, Craig K. Pain expression and cry. Pain. 1987. 28, 395-410.

6. Dale J. A multidimensional study of infants' responses to painful stimuli. Paediatric Nursing. 1986, 12, 1, 27-31.

7. Brown L. Physiological responses to cutaneous pain in neonates. Neonatal Network. 1987, 18-22.

8. Williamson P, Williamson M. Physiological stress reduction by a local anaesthetic during newborn circumcision. Pediatrics. 1983, 71, 1, 36-40.

9. Harpin V, Rutter N. Development of emotional sweating in the newborn infant. Archives of Disease in Childhood. 1982. 57, 691-5.

10. Gauvain-Piquard A. Comment reconnaitre la douleur d'un enfant. Revue de l'infirmière. 1987. 15, 19-24.

11. Sparshott M. Pain and the Special Care Baby Unit. Nursing Times. 1989. 85, 41, 61-64.

12. Sparshott M. Creating a home for babies in hospital. Paediatric Nursing. 1991, 3, 8, 20-22.

FURTHER READING

There are many physiology texts which are useful to nurses. We have suggested some that you might find useful, but this is not an exhaustive list.

ALEXANDER J.I. & HILL R.G. (1987) Postoperative Pain Control. Blackwell Scientific, Oxford. A useful text for people with an interest in postoperative care.

BERNE R.M. & LEVY M.N. (1990) Principles of Physiology. C. V. Mosby Co. Wolfe, London. A comprehensive reference text.

GREEN J.H. (1989) An Introduction to Human Physiology (4th Edition). Oxford University Press, Oxford. This is a short and approachable book.

HINCHCLIFFE S. & MONTAGUE S. (1988) Physiology for Nursing Practice. Bailliere Tindall. This book gives a more detailed description and includes explanations of some of the changes in function that occur in illness.

HOSKING J. & WELCHEW E. (1985) Postoperative Pain: Understanding its Nature and How to Treat it. Faber and Faber, London. A useful text for hospital based care.

HUBBARD J.L. & MECHAN D.J. (1991) Physiology for Health Studies. Churchill Livingstone. Colleagues have described this as "an excellent book" which is appropriate when you already have a basic understanding of physiology.

MACKENNA B.R. & CALLENDER R. (1990) Illustrated Physiology. Churchill Livingstone. This book uses a diagrammatic format to explain the ways the body functions. If you like short descriptions this might suit you.

MARIEB E.N. (1993) Human Anatomy & Physiology. Benjamin Cummings Publishing. A good reference source.

NEAL M.J. (1992) Medical Pharmacology at a Glance (2nd Edition). Blackwell Scientific, Oxford. Excellent text, but requires some detailed knowledge of physiology.

PUNTILLO K.A. (1991) Pain in the Critically Ill - Assessment and Management. Aspen Publishers, Maryland, USA. A comprehensive reference text.

RANG H.P. & DALE M.M. (1987) Pharmacology. Longman. A comprehensive reference text.

Royal College of Surgeons of England and College of Anaesthetists. (September 1990) Pain after Surgery: Report of Working Party. A useful informative document.

SOFAER B. (1992) Pain: A Handbook for Nurses (New Edition). Harper and Row. An excellent text for all carers.

WILKINSON R. (1992) 'Pulmonary artery pressure monitoring'. Nursing Standard 25, July 8/Volume 6/Number 42. A practical account of this important clinical procedure and its physiological basis.